THE COMPLETE PTSD RECOVERY PROCESS:

A Life-Changing Step-by-Step Blueprint to Triumph over Trauma and Reclaim Your Life with Tapping (EFT)

Copyright and Disclosures

Copyright © 2019
by Sure Path LLC

All rights reserved. No part of this publication may be reproduced, distributed, or transmitted in any form or by any means, including photocopying, recording, or other electronic or mechanical methods, without the prior written permission of the publisher, except in the case of brief quotations embodied in reviews and certain other noncommercial uses permitted by copyright law.

While all attempts have been made to verify the information provided in this publication, neither the author nor the publisher assumes any responsibility for errors, omissions, or contrary interpretations on the subject matter herein. This book is for entertainment purposes only. The views expressed are those of the author alone and should not be taken as expert instruction or commands. The reader is responsible for his or her own actions. Adherence to all applicable laws and regulations, including international, federal, state, and local governing professional licensing, business practices, advertising, and all other aspects of doing business in the US, Canada, or any other jurisdiction is the sole responsibility of the reader or purchaser. Neither the author nor the publisher assumes any responsibility or liability whatsoever on behalf of the purchaser or reader of these materials.

FREE PTSD CHECKUP

Welcome! I'm glad you're here.

As a special bonus for you, I've created a free PTSD checkup. This test will give you an accurate measure of how you're doing with PTSD. Measuring is a helpful place to start on your healing journey. It gives you a real baseline for measuring progress later.

Ready to get a *real* sense of how you're doing? Go to www.bit.ly/PTSDHealing for your free PTSD checkup. Type in keyword: PTSD checkup.

A QUICK NOTE ON RESOURCES THROUGHOUT THIS BOOK

This book is packed with helpful resources like the PTSD checkup above, cheat sheets, handouts, videos, and other helpful tools. These resources will all be delivered via Facebook Messenger. In each section of the book where resources are available, you'll find a keyword to type into Facebook Messenger to retrieve them. Type in the designated keyword, and you'll immediately get access to the relevant links and tools. Note: retype them exactly as they appear in the book.

Additionally, you can access Facebook Messenger resources at www.bit.ly/PTSDHealing. To join other folks who are working to resolve their trauma and PTSD through the tools and processes in this book, join the Transforming Trauma: The Secrets of Healing Trauma + PTSD For Good Facebook Group at http://bit.ly/PTSDFBGroup and Like the David Redbord Facebook Page at http://bit.ly/PTSDFBPage.

CONTENTS

Introduction 1

   Why Are We Talking about Tapping? 4

CHAPTER 1:
The Path to Reclaiming Your Life and
Triumphing over Trauma—The Healing Trauma
Blueprint 10

   In This Chapter 11

   The Event 12

   Trauma 12

   Trauma in the Brain 13

   Trauma in the Physical Body 14

   Trauma and the Emotions 15

   Trauma in the Energy Body 16

   The Impact of Trauma on the Body 17

   Posttraumatic Growth 20

   Clearing the Charge 21

How Can We Clear the Charge? 21

Why Tapping for Trauma? 24

How Tapping Works 25

Short-Term Strategies 27

Long-Term Strategies 29

Bringing in the Positive 29

What Happens as We Clear the Trauma? 30

Self-Care 32

Mindfulness 34

Additional Thoughts about Self-Care 37

Managing Daily Emotions 38

Healing Trauma Blueprint 45

What It Really Looks Like 46

CHAPTER 2:
Conquering the Sadness, Anxiety, Depression, Anger, Fear, and Overwhelm—How to Use Tapping to Manage Daily Emotions **50**

In This Chapter 50

Tapping Overview 50

Tapping Sequence Part One 55

Practicing the Tapping Points 55

The Two Secret Techniques: Breath and Sound 58

Practicing the Tapping Points with Sound and Breath 59

Two Types of Tapping: Additive and Reductive 63

The First Half of the Reductive Tapping Practice Round..67

Practicing the 9-Gamut Procedure 71

The Second Half of the Reductive Practice Round............72

What Do You Do If You Still Have Some Intensity? 76

Additive Tapping..77

The First Half of the Additive Practice Round 79

The Second Half of the Additive Practice Round..............84

When to Use Tapping...89

Considerations..90

CHAPTER 3:
Stop the Nightmares, Intrusive Thoughts, and Triggers for Good—How to Use Tapping to Drastically Reduce PTSD at Its Core So You Can Move On with Your Life.. 93

In This Chapter 93

Trauma and Safety..94

A Biological and Emotional Perspective............................94

An Energetic Perspective...95

Trauma in the Chakras 96

Trauma and Addiction 97

The Most Important Reason to Create Safety: The Window of Tolerance 97

How to Create Safety: Resourcing 98

Guided Meditation 99

Resourcing Meditation Practice Process 102

Making a List of Your Traumatic Memories 106

Tell the Story: Up to 3/10 Intensity 111

Use Tapping 111

Tapping through the Remaining Feelings 113

Continuing to Tell the Story: Up to a 10/10 Intensity 116

Tapping through This Intensity 117

Go through This for All Memories on the List from Most to Least Intense 120

Bringing in the Positive with Additive Tapping 121

Additive Tapping ideas 122

Additive Tapping Practice Process: Safety 123

What Does This Mean for PTSD Symptoms? 128

PTSD Symptoms: An Energetic Perspective 129

Bill's Case Study: Before and After 130

Bill's Scores: Before and After 131

Resource List 136

Works Cited 140

INTRODUCTION

Dear Reader,

This book was created as a guide to help you resolve your trauma at the root and to care for yourself daily. It is my privilege to be able to share this with you. At this point, I've worked with hundreds of clients to create healing around all manner of different issues: physical, mental, emotional, and spiritual. I've facilitated workshops around the country and worked with clients across the world.

I wasn't always in a position to help others—to share with them the overflow from my own full cup. There was a time when my cup was quite empty. When I was a teenager, I was diagnosed with depression and anxiety, and I was suicidal. I attempted to kill myself five times in my teen years. The burden of shame I felt within myself was so heavy. I was in constant internal emotional pain all the time. I ranged between feeling numbness, anger, and despair. I numbed out because I didn't want to deal with the pain. I wanted to die because I wanted the pain to end. I didn't have very many friendships as a teenager because I didn't like myself. In fact, I downright hated myself. If I didn't like myself, why would someone else?

As I entered college, I started to desire something else. As I embarked on my first master's degree program, that desire grew to a point where I *had* to act on it. I wanted to feel better, I wanted to feel more connected to myself, I wanted to connect more with others, and I wanted to find my own answers. I wanted to have fulfilling, meaningful relationships with people, romantically and in friendships. I didn't know it at the time, but that was going to take work. Not work in the sense of boring, monotonous tasks with little reward but rather a willingness to face my own internal demons head-on, not shy away, and reap the massive rewards of doing so.

When I started, I was disconnected from myself because I had numbed out—because I had distanced myself from myself. If I was disconnected from myself, I certainly couldn't connect with anyone else. That's like offering to share food with someone when I didn't bring any. There is nothing to share.

As far as answers go, I certainly couldn't rely on what I'd learned in school or through religion or my upbringing, as those answers had gotten me where I was, and that wasn't some place I liked being. It was constant, ongoing suffering and ongoing effort to avoid feeling the suffering. I avoided my reality through video games, books, and television. I became addicted to video games. I played them for eight hours a day for three years during my teen years to escape the pain I was feeling.

If I was going to do the things I wanted, feel better, connect with myself and others, and find my own answers, all that had to change. I started going to spiritual meetups where I lived in

New Orleans. I got certified in Reiki, Pranic Healing, Psych-K, and other things. I got trained in a variety of techniques, such as authentic leadership, compassionate communication, breathwork, inner child work, and tapping. I tried *tons* of things. Each of those things helped me in its own way. Each contributed to my path toward wellness. I haven't stopped either. I just finished my second master's degree in clinical mental health counseling.

As you can see, I have traveled *many* different paths to arrive where I am now. I have traveled many different roads for the last ten years to accomplish the healing within myself that I have presently achieved. As a child, I had been in therapy from ages eight to seventeen. I had four different therapists. Only with the fourth did I experience some benefit. Still, none of it touched the deeper layers. None of it created lasting change.

I must own my role in that, though, as you must in your own healing process. I, at the time I saw those therapists, was not willing to go deep. I was not willing to face my own emotions because I thought they were so strong that they would kill me if I did. I have faced them many times since, and not only am I still alive, but my threshold to tolerate my own intensity and that of others has also drastically increased as a result of my willingness to face my own stuff.

When I started this path, there was no road map, there was no path. So dear reader, I have created this book to save you the tens of thousands of dollars and years I've spent in pursuit of my own healing. I have traveled the unexplored territory and created for you a map with clear signposts and specific directions. This way, you don't have to get lost, sidetracked, derailed, or pick up a case of yellow fever unexpectedly in your travels. It is with great care and love that I offer this to you as your map as you pursue your own healing and release the burden that *you've* been carrying. Be warned, though: the road is ongoing. Healing is a process of going deeper and deeper. That said, if you follow the steps and principles in this book, you can experience lasting change.

Why Are We Talking about Tapping?

When some people think of tapping, they think of someone making a rather irritating noise with their fingers, feet, a pen, or a pencil. I'm going to talk to you about another type of tapping called the Emotional Freedom Techniques or EFT. It's a holistic healing method where we physically tap on the meridian points in our body with our fingertips while verbalizing what we're working on out loud, so our subconscious gets on board with our healing as well. If that sounds a bit vague and confusing right now, don't worry. It will be clarified in detail in chapters 2 and 3.

Why are we talking about tapping? Of the myriad healing techniques that I have been certified and trained in, tapping is one of the most successful for working with trauma and post-traumatic stress disorder (PTSD). From a mental health standpoint, tapping could be compared to eye movement desensitization reprocessing (EMDR), cognitive processing therapy, and exposure therapy in that they are all techniques to help integrate the trauma you've experienced. The key difference is tapping is something you can do yourself. You don't have to go see a therapist for years or spend tons of money. You can do it yourself with the instructions I've offered here in this book. This is tremendously empowering. You can take your healing into your own hands rather than relying on someone else to do it or facilitate it for you; you remain in control.

Tapping also has some very impressive research data behind it for things like PTSD, anxiety, depression, phobias, pain, and addiction. So we're not just hanging out talking about woo-woo space nonsense. We're talking about a discipline that originates in Chinese medicine, which has been practiced for thousands of years and has been backed by a ton of research studies.

In one such study led by Dawson Church (2013), 59 veterans with PTSD were divided into two groups. Half (30) received six sessions of tapping, and half (29) were placed on a waitlist. After the six sessions, 90 percent of the 30 veterans who had done the tapping sessions were no longer diagnosable with PTSD. Only 4 percent of the waitlist group were also no longer diagnosable. Six months later, 80 percent of those 30 veterans who had done tapping were still no longer diagnosable with PTSD. The veterans who had received the tapping also had significant decreases in anxiety and depression, and a 41 percent decrease in physical pain on average. When you heal trauma, anxiety and depression tend to improve as well, according to the research (National Collaborating Centre for Mental Health, 2005).

As I began to do the deeper work of healing my traumatic memories, my anxiety and depression started to improve. I watched my depression go from once a month to once every two months, to once every six months, and now very rarely. My anxiety and hypervigilance have also drastically decreased. I've witnessed this in my clients as well.

So how did I discover tapping? I had studied, trained, and certified in several techniques as I mentioned in the first introduction. I had begun practicing on myself, then with people I knew, and eventually I opened my own healing practice. I worked with many different people over the years that I maintained my in-person practice. I also had the privilege of working in an office with many different practitioners doing all kinds of different healing techniques. It was there that I first encountered tapping. I was skeptical at first. Why did I need *another* technique? I already had so many. Besides that, it surely looked strange seeing someone tap on their body. My path had other things in mind, though.

I won a ticket to an event with a slew of workshops, and one was for tapping. I sat with about 30 other people as the facilitator lead us through a tapping process about our parental wounding. I cried, and when I looked around at the other people, many of them were crying too. I could feel the big emotional release that I had. I knew there was something special here. I went home and studied material from Gary Craig, one of the founders of tapping. I learned to facilitate it for myself, then I began to practice it with clients, and I saw miraculous results.

What else do you call it when you can sit with someone for 60 or so minutes and watch as the trauma they've been carrying from a severe car accident no longer affects them by the time they leave the office? A miracle. Another time, I had a client who had never done any kind of holistic or alternative healing drive eight hours to see me at the urging of her daughter. Talk about pressure to deliver results. She was suffering from substantial circulation issues and experienced physical pain as a result. She reported feeling a pain level of 8/10 on her wrist and 10/10 on her lower leg. We began to tap on her memories of when the pain was the absolute worst. When we had finished several rounds of tapping and an hour or so had passed, I checked in with her about the pain on a scale from 0 to 10. She replied, "There's no pain? There's no pain . . . there's no pain!" She couldn't believe that the pain was no longer there. As you can see, tapping can yield substantial results, which are backed by the research.

I had reached a wall. You see, it was one thing for people to come into my office and have me guide them through a healing process. I wanted to empower people to heal themselves on their own time. Doing that was easier said than done. As I mentioned in the introduction, there was no road map I could hand to people to say, "Here you go. Now you'll be able to take care of this yourself," in any kind of systematic way. I wanted to create something that would empower people to take their healing into their own hands and achieve the results they wanted.

Every day I take a walk on a lovely trail near my house. It helps me to process what's on my mind and move my energy so it doesn't stagnate. Plus, the exercise is beneficial too. As I walk, I often have ideas that come in because I'm not distracted by my phone or the television or anything else that we use to take ourselves out of the present in our current time. I make an effort to stay present and not do anything else.

One day as I walked, I had a series of ideas come in. I was going to create a course. The course would look this way and contain these modules and processes. When I thought about who this course would work best for, folks with trauma and PTSD came to mind, as I had seen the benefits for myself and for my clients too. I remembered that I had seen them in the material I had studied as well. I built that course.

I wanted to make the material even more accessible. I wanted to empower even more people. So I created this book, distilling down the core elements of the course into a digestible format that can be read in one afternoon, and realistically implemented within a month with major results. It can further be implemented until you've cleared the emotional charge from the majority of your traumatic memories.

Why trauma? I have found that trauma is at the root of most suffering. You'll learn more about some research-backed examples of that in chapter 1 (Felitti et al., 1998). If you can alleviate that suffering, I have found that more joy, freedom, and peace naturally fill in the space where the trauma once lived. The more trauma you clear out, the more joy, freedom, and peace come in. That's what I have seen in my clients, myself, and what the research shows too (Tedeschi & Calhoun, 1996).

If you can get the trauma out of the way by integrating and releasing it rather than fighting against it, it primes you to enjoy the rest of your life. This book is here to give you the tools to integrate and release the trauma that has been weighing you down so you can move on with your life. As you'll see, the main trauma healing process is done through tapping, and I've incorporated and offered other accessible skills that I've found very effective for myself and my clients to help you care for yourself and manage your emotions on a daily basis. Even when you heal as much of your trauma as you can, life doesn't somehow stop. It goes on, and emotions, pleasant or otherwise, will continue to come and go. In this book, I've given you some of the key tools to work with whatever you encounter within and outside yourself.

Remember to treat yourself with kindness as you go through your healing process. Don't rush yourself and don't put pressure on yourself to be further along than where you are. That pressure adds to the burden on your system and keeps you from healing as effectively. Instead, acknowledge where you are in your healing process and move forward from there at your own pace. This book is a road map. It doesn't come with a speedometer to tell you how fast you *should* be going. I can assure you not to worry. Your whole identity isn't suddenly going to change. Get the suffering out of the way progressively, and more and more well-being comes in to replace it.

In support of you finding your way back to the health and well-being that is your birthright,

David

CHAPTER 1:

THE PATH TO RECLAIMING YOUR LIFE AND TRIUMPHING OVER TRAUMA—THE HEALING TRAUMA BLUEPRINT

Rumi said, "Your task is not to seek for love but merely to seek and find all the barriers within yourself that you have built against it."

I find that trauma is arguably the largest barrier that we have within us. It keeps us from receiving love and allowing love into our lives. This trauma can occur on multiple levels. One level may be in response to trauma. We've hardened ourselves because we don't feel safe to be vulnerable. Trauma can impact our self-esteem. We feel unworthy of receiving love because of what's happened to us. Rumi is suggesting that, rather than seeking love itself, love exists. If you are aware of the barriers within yourself and work with them, you can allow love in. The purpose of this book is to help you get the barriers caused by trauma out of the way so you can live a more enjoyable, fulfilled life—one that includes more love.

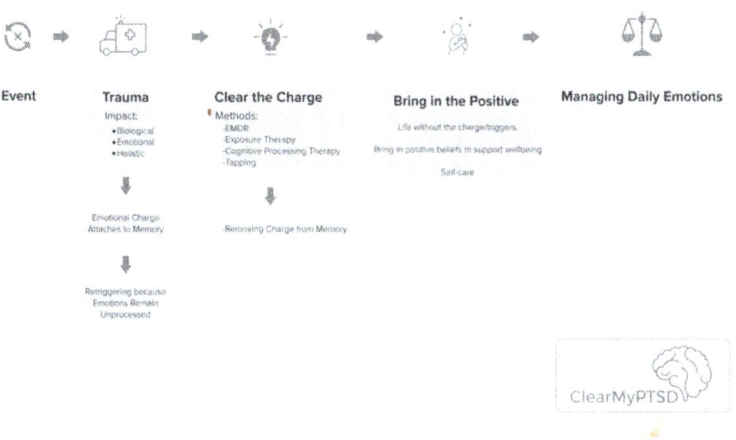

Figure 1. The healing trauma blueprint.

This is the healing trauma blueprint (figure 1). Trauma is a response to an event that registers in our system. An emotional charge attaches to the memory, and retriggering is happening because the emotions remain unprocessed. We work with trauma by clearing the charge. Once we clear the charge, we create more space internally, which allows us to bring in more positive beliefs and well-being in general. On a daily basis, we're working with managing our emotions and self-care.

In This Chapter

In this chapter, we're going to look at what makes an event traumatic. We'll discuss trauma from a biological, holistic, and emotional perspective. Following this, we'll look at clearing the emotional charge and check out some techniques: eye movement desensitization and reprocessing, exposure therapy, cognitive processing therapy, and tapping. Then we will get a sense of what life is like without the charge and how we use self-care for the upkeep of our well-being. Lastly, we'll explore some strategies for managing our daily emotions.

The Event

Let's take a look at the event. An event could be anything like a car accident, sexual assault, natural disaster, or childhood wound. There's a wide range of events that can cause trauma. Realistically, any event can cause trauma. It's just a matter of how our system processes an event. The event by itself is not yet trauma. If a hundred people experience a car accident, some portion of those people will be able to bounce back and continue going about their lives. Another proportion of those folks will have something in their system that gets stuck. That is trauma.

Trauma

Trauma is anything that we encounter that is beyond the capacity of our mind-body system to effectively process. Trauma can be looked at through three lenses: biological, emotional, and energetic. If our mind-body system could process it effectively, it wouldn't get stuck, and we wouldn't have trauma.

Trauma in the Brain
(Biological Perspective)

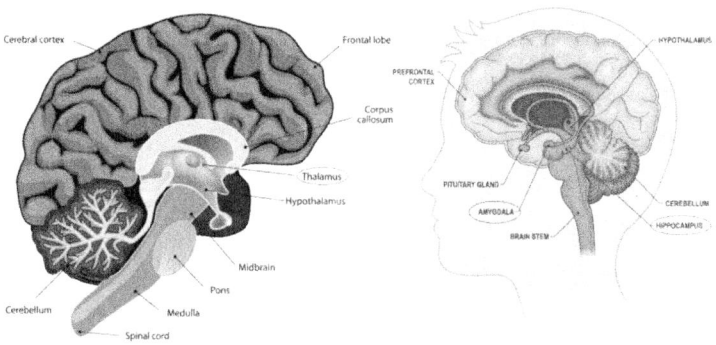

Figure 2. How the brain processes trauma.

Let's look at trauma from a brain perspective (figure 2). Earlier, we talked about some examples of possible traumatic events. Anything that is happening in our environment, whether it's a car accident or an earthquake or just eating lunch, is data taken in by our brain through the senses. This data arrives at a part of the brain called the thalamus (van der Kolk, 2014). Anything we're seeing, hearing, touching, or tasting is taken in through the thalamus where it's filtered to another part of the brain called the amygdala.

The amygdala is the emotional processing center of the brain. It looks at this incoming data and labels it accordingly (van der Kolk, 2014). If it looks like a sad thing that happened, the amygdala puts a sad stamp on it. If it's an event that feels mostly like anger, the amygdala puts an angry stamp on it. After that, the brain puts it in the hippocampus, which is the memory storage center of your brain. There it can be stored and retrieved as needed.

A similar process happens with trauma. The brains of people who experience trauma are also taking in the same sensory information through the thalamus. Afterward, it goes to the amygdala. The amygdala then looks at the information and encodes it with the appropriate emotional label: angry, sad, fear, shame, guilt, doubt—whatever the feelings are. As a result of the perceived intensity of the emotion contained in the memory, the memory/information doesn't move into long-term storage. It hangs out in this part of the brain where it remains unprocessed. Since it's unprocessed, it's very easy for it to get retriggered. If another experience that comes into your awareness gets processed by the thalamus, arrives at the amygdala, and reminds us of this unprocessed event, it leads to a trigger. A trigger is a disproportionate emotional reaction to whatever the current situation is. Meaning if the situation seems to warrant a 2/10 for anger, but you're at a 10/10, you've probably been triggered. In other words, the size of the reaction is huge compared to what is actually justified by the situation.

That's why certain sights, sounds, and smells can retrigger us. They're getting filtered in through the thalamus, stamped and labeled in the amygdala, and touching on the unprocessed stuff that's hanging around that area.

Trauma in the Physical Body

Trauma and stress can also be stored in the physical body. That's why sometimes people have physical symptoms like tremors, shaking, pain, and nausea (van der Kolk, 2014). These can actually be results of trauma in the body.

Trauma and the Emotions

Trauma is when the emotional charge we experience from an event exceeds our threshold to tolerate it (Ogden, 2006). I find the image of an overflowing cup helpful for this concept (figure 3). If the cup could contain all the water being poured in, it wouldn't overflow. If our system could handle the emotional charge, it wouldn't result in trauma. You can see that this cup is not able to contain the quantity of water that's coming in. In very much the same way, when our system is unable to deal with the intensity of an emotional charge, it lands in the system as trauma. If that emotional charge doesn't exceed our ability to tolerate it, it doesn't become trauma. Without that quality of exceeding our threshold, we're left with just an event. Without this substantial emotional charge, we just have an event. Without this overflow, we just have a cup with water in it.

Going Deeper with Emotions

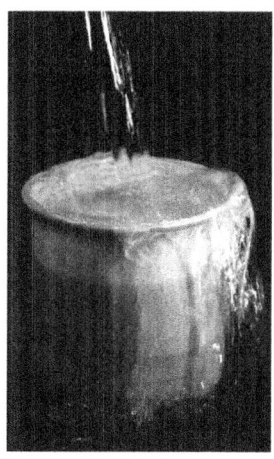

Figure 3. The overflowing cup.

Let's go deeper for a moment and look at why some folks have nightmares, intrusive thoughts, and triggers. It's because there's an unprocessed emotional charge stuck in the system. With all three of these issues, your subconscious mind is trying to find resolution about what happened. It wants to deal with the water that's overflowing from the cup. It's bringing these things to your attention through nightmares, intrusive thoughts, and retriggering. You can think about this as a call for help (Riedl, 2006). It's as if your subconscious mind is raising its hand and asking you for your attention. There's something that needs your attention here, and this is how your system is pointing it out to you.

Trauma in the Energy Body

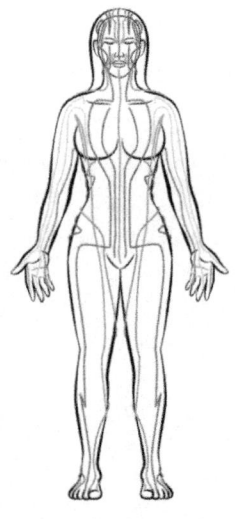

Figure 4. The meridian system.

We have a meridian system that flows through our body (figure 4). Energy is constantly moving through this system. All disease from this perspective is caused by a block in the flow of energy through this system. It doesn't matter whether that disease is physical, mental, emotional, or spiritual. There's some obstruction in the system. Just like before where we saw that stuff is stuck hanging out by the amygdala, it's very much the same thing here. The energy that would normally flow through the system freely gets stuck (Gallo, 2004). The energy is no longer flowing properly, causing us to be retriggered and potentially leading to physical health effects.

The Impact of Trauma on the Body

From 1995 to 1997 a survey was conducted by Kaiser Permanente, one of the biggest health care systems in California. Through data gathered from 17,000 people concerning adverse childhood experiences, researchers began to notice a pattern. Many of their patients who were morbidly obese also seemed to have substantial trauma in their childhood.

Adverse Childhood Experience (ACE) Questionnaire
Finding your ACE Score ra hbr 10 24 06

While you were growing up, during your first 18 years of life:

1. Did a parent or other adult in the household **often** …
   Swear at you, insult you, put you down, or humiliate you?
       or
   Act in a way that made you afraid that you might be physically hurt?
       Yes No   If yes enter 1 _____

2. Did a parent or other adult in the household **often** …
   Push, grab, slap, or throw something at you?
       or
   Ever hit you so hard that you had marks or were injured?
       Yes No   If yes enter 1 _____

3. Did an adult or person at least 5 years older than you **ever**…
   Touch or fondle you or have you touch their body in a sexual way?
       or
   Try to or actually have oral, anal, or vaginal sex with you?
       Yes No   If yes enter 1 _____

4. Did you **often** feel that …
   No one in your family loved you or thought you were important or special?
       or
   Your family didn't look out for each other, feel close to each other, or support each other?
       Yes No   If yes enter 1 _____

5. Did you **often** feel that …
   You didn't have enough to eat, had to wear dirty clothes, and had no one to protect you?
       or
   Your parents were too drunk or high to take care of you or take you to the doctor if you needed it?
       Yes No   If yes enter 1 _____

6. Were your parents **ever** separated or divorced?
       Yes No   If yes enter 1 _____

7. Was your mother or stepmother:
   Often pushed, grabbed, slapped, or had something thrown at her?
       or
   Sometimes or often kicked, bitten, hit with a fist, or hit with something hard?
       or
   Ever repeatedly hit over at least a few minutes or threatened with a gun or knife?
       Yes No   If yes enter 1 _____

8. Did you live with anyone who was a problem drinker or alcoholic or who used street drugs?
       Yes No   If yes enter 1 _____

9. Was a household member depressed or mentally ill or did a household member attempt suicide?
       Yes No   If yes enter 1 _____

10. Did a household member go to prison?
        Yes No   If yes enter 1 _____

Now add up your "Yes" answers: _____ This is your ACE Score

Figure 5. The adverse childhood experience questionnaire.

Exercise

This is the Adverse Childhood Experience Study (ACES) created by the Kaiser Permanente researchers (figure 5).

1. Get a piece of paper and jot down your answers to these questions. If you answer yes to question one, mark yes. If you answer yes to question two, mark yes and so on.
2. When you're done with these questions, count how many times you answered yes.

Go to www.bit.ly/PTSDHealing to access a printable version of the ACE questionnaire. Use Messenger keyword: ACE questionnaire.

Impact of ACES	
Alcoholism and alcohol abuse	Early initiation of sexual activity
Chronic obstructive pulmonary disease	Adolescent pregnancy
Depression	Risk of sexual violence
Fetal death	Poor academic achievement
Health-related quality of life	Heart attack
Illicit drug use	Asthma
Ischemic heart disease	Mental distress
Liver disease	Depression
Poor work performance	Disability
Financial stress	Reported income
Risk for intimate partner violence	Unemployment
Multiple sexual partners	Lowered educational attainment

Sexually transmitted diseases	Coronary heart disease
Smoking	Stroke
Suicide attempts	Diabetes
Unintended pregnancies	Early initiation of smoking

Figure 6. Health and life outcomes associated with adverse childhood experiences (ACEs).

These are the potential impacts of those adverse childhood experiences in life according to the data (figure 6). The more adverse childhood experiences you have, the more likely you are to have these hurdles in life (Felitti et al., 1998). There is a dose-response relationship: the impact is directly proportionate to the number of ACEs that you have been exposed to. If you have one adverse childhood experience, you are somewhat more likely to have these symptoms. If you have more than one, the likelihood of experiencing these issues increases. Each of the experiences discussed in the survey directly increases the likelihood of having more trauma later in life.

Posttraumatic Growth

We've said earlier that some folks experience trauma and they bounce back immediately. Then there are some folks that experience trauma and afterward end up with some distress and confusion. For the latter group, they try and make sense of what happened. Why did this happen to me? Why did this happen in my life? What does it mean? For those people that end up with that distress and confusion, there is a process that happens as they go through their healing journey.

As they come out the other side, they can often experience posttraumatic growth. Posttraumatic growth is when there are positive changes in their ability to appreciate life and the things that are happening in life, the quality of their relationships and connections with others, and their ability to see new possibilities in life (Tedeschi & Calhoun, 1996). Having now been through the event, they're able to appreciate life more and see new possibilities in it. They can feel stronger and more resilient. Their self-confidence increases, their sense of well-being increases, and they may feel more connected to the universe and their sense of spirituality. These are the benefits of going through this trauma healing process.

Clearing the Charge

How do we go about the trauma healing process? We create safety, and then we clear the emotional charge around what happened. Earlier, we've said that the event plus the emotional charge is what leads to trauma. If we remove the emotional charge from the trauma, all we're left with is the event. The charge is no longer there, and the trauma becomes a memory. Without the charge, the memory can be thought of or discussed without getting triggered.

How Can We Clear the Charge?

Earlier, I used the phrases unprocessed and processed. When I say processed, I'm referring to a memory which has had the emotional charge cleared and integrated. We're working with the memory. We're actively using some process that's going to help us to clear the charge.

An unprocessed memory is one that we haven't worked with. To go back to the biological brain perspective, the memory is still hanging out by the amygdala impacting us. To go back to the energy system perspective, since the memory is unprocessed stuck energy in the system, it continues to cause us distress. When we process something, we're moving the energy through our system to a point where it's no longer impacting us from this perspective.

When we process it from a biological perspective, we're removing the emotional charge which allows the memory to move from the amygdala to the hippocampus, the memory storage center in the brain.

Below are four different techniques for processing these memories. First, there's prolonged exposure—repeating the story of the event or trauma many times ("Prolonged Exposure," 2017). By repeating the experience many times, we become desensitized to it, and it no longer affects us. It's almost as if you have a job that's very repetitive and very tedious. Eventually you stop paying attention to what you're doing because it's in your subconscious memory, and you can do it just by rote without having to think about it. If you repeat the trauma many, many times, eventually you will get to a point where repeating it doesn't bring up anxiety and stress for you anymore.

Cognitive processing therapy is another method which involves changing how we think about and process the event or trauma ("Cognitive Processing," 2017). We're shifting our thoughts and mentality about it. By changing how we feel about it, we're changing how it impacts us daily.

We also have eye movement and desensitization reprocessing, also called EMDR ("Eye Movement," 2017). With this method, we're stimulating both hemispheres of the brain while we're thinking about what happened. We do that by moving our eyes back and forth, through listening to a sound on headphones that goes back and forth from one ear to the other, or by holding things in our hands that vibrate alternately. By stimulating both hemispheres of the brain, we're bringing more of the brain online to help us process the trauma. The idea behind EMDR is that the whole brain wasn't online when this event happened, and as a result, things got stuck as we've been seeing. If we can bring more of the brain online and reprocess what happened, then we can clear the charge.

Lastly, there is a method called emotional freedom techniques (EFT or tapping). Tapping combines elements of all three of the above methods and moves the emotional charge through the system (Solomon, 2007). By physically tapping on the meridian points in our body, we are moving the energy through the system and allowing the system to come back to a state of well-being. Also, with tapping, what we're doing is we're very consciously bringing love and acceptance to whatever it was that happened and how we feel about it now. Through that love and acceptance, the emotions integrate, and the charge clears.

Success Rates for Healing PTSD

Method	Success rate
Prolonged exposure Cognitive processing therapy Eye movement desensitization reprocessing (EMDR)	Up to 78.3%*
Emotional Freedom Techniques (tapping)	Up to 90%*

Figure 7. Success rates for different PTSD treatment methods.

Typically, prolonged exposure has a success rate up to 65 percent (Kar, 2011). Cognitive processing therapy has about the same success rate as EMDR (Kar, 2011). EMDR has up to a 78.3 percent success rate (Kar, 2011). Tapping, according to the data, has up to a 90 percent success rate (Church et al., 2018).

Why Tapping for Trauma?

Situation/type of trauma	PTSD research results
Veterans	90% no longer diagnosable with PTSD after 6 hours
Earthquake survivors	72% decrease in symptom severity
Sexual assault	Significant improvement
Abuse survivors	Dramatically reduced avoidance and intrusive thoughts

Figure 8. Examples of study results for tapping and PTSD.

Here are some of the different results from published studies on the benefits of tapping for different types of trauma (figure 8). On the left, there are different types of traumatic experiences:

veterans who have been exposed to war, earthquake survivors, sexual assault survivors, and abuse survivors. After six hours of tapping, 90 percent of veterans were no longer diagnosable with PTSD. Likewise with earthquake survivors, there was a 72 percent decrease in symptom severity after tapping (Gurret, Caufour, Palmer-Hoffman, & Church, 2012). In regard to sexual assault, researchers found a significant improvement (Nemiro & Papworth, 2015). For abuse survivors who had childhood wounding and childhood trauma, researchers saw dramatically reduced avoidance and intrusive thoughts (Church, Piña, Reategui, & Brooks, 2012).

How Tapping Works

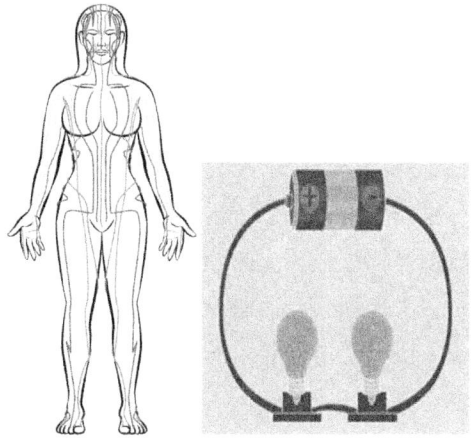

Figure 9. The meridian system as a circuit.

Think about this energy system like a circuit, where a battery connects to a light bulb with a wire (figure 9). When that wire is connected, the light turns on. If there's anything that's interrupting this flow of energy from the battery to the light bulb, the light bulb can't turn on (Solomon, 2007). The trauma disrupts the flow of energy through the system. So our light, our well-being, can't turn on to the same degree that it would if that disruption to the flow of energy wasn't there. With tapping, we are clearing that disruption, clearing that emotional charge, which allows the energy to flow properly.

What Does All That Mean?

If we clear the emotional charge from our traumatic memories, they won't get erased. It's not like what happened never happened to us. It's that we can now recall the memories without the emotional charge. Without that charge, we can go about our lives with fewer triggers, fewer nightmares, and fewer intrusive thoughts or even none at all (Church, Piña, Reategui, & Brooks, 2012).

How Do We Make That Happen?

We have short-term strategies, and we have long-term strategies. EMDR, tapping, cognitive processing therapy, and exposure therapy are long-term strategies. We set aside time so we can work with the memory to create change that lasts long term. As a result of the work, the charge is no longer there, so we can have increased well-being for the rest of our lives. It can take several hours, weeks, or even a few months to create this lasting long-term charge.

Short-term strategies are how we work with ourselves and our emotions in the moment. While we're doing the deeper work for clearing the charge, we use short-term strategies to work with ourselves and our emotions daily. We continue to use these strategies daily even after we finish the trauma healing work.

Short-Term Strategies

There are two types of short-term strategies: internal and external. Internal strategies start with noticing our emotional and body-based experiences. Our body has so much information to tell us if we start paying attention to it as do our emotions. Culturally, what I find is that there's a lot of emphasis on the mind. The mind is given priority over the emotions and the body. Yet, if we can bring the body and the emotions online, we can start to notice what information they have for us in addition to the information we get from the mind. Conversely, if we're not aware of what our emotions and our body are telling us, we are operating at a deficit. We don't have that information, so we can't use it in our healing process.

Short-term strategy includes becoming more literate in our emotions and our bodily sensations. Examples include noticing when we have a tightness in the belly, clenched muscles, or a tight jaw. Each of these things is usually indicative of an underlying emotional experience.

We can work with our mental, emotional, and bodily experiences using different methods. We can use mindfulness and specific tools to integrate the underlying emotions. Below are the tools we use to work with what's going on inside ourselves.

We want to be able to work and communicate with others effectively. This is where external strategies come in. First, we notice what's happening internally in terms of our emotions and our bodily sensations. This is what's happening inside ourselves. As we go about our lives, we're often interacting with other people, so we want to be able to communicate with them effectively about what's happening inside. We want to be able to cultivate the skills to be able to voice our feelings and needs to others. We want to cultivate the ability and the willingness to ask for what we want and need (Rosenberg, 2003).

For example, if you're experiencing a trigger, maybe you need some space to process it safely. You want to get comfortable noticing that and then asking for what you need around that request for space.

Another facet of external strategy is our willingness to take responsibility for our role in interactions (Weinhold & Weinhold, 2017). For example, when we get triggered, it is a lot easier and convenient to be unkind. In this example, we would want to take responsibility for how we're treating others and how we're showing up in these different interactions. If we take responsibility for how we're showing up, ask for what we need, and get comfortable voicing our feelings and needs to others, we can create much healthier and more connected relationships. We notice what's happening inside, and then we cultivate the skills to be able to communicate that with people outside ourselves.

Long-Term Strategies

Long-term strategies are how we clear the emotional charge from the original memories, and I recommend tapping for that (Gallo, 2007). I'm recommending that in large part because the research shows how impactful it can be, and I love the fact that it's something you can do yourself. You probably need some guidance and instruction on how to do it. However, once you know how, it's something that you can do yourself at home when you have time. I find it really empowering. I really like tapping for those two reasons: the research backing and the independence.

Bringing in the Positive

We looked at the traumatic event, and we then looked at clearing the emotional charge from the trauma so that the trauma just becomes an event, a memory that happened. In the process of doing that, what happens is we clear some internal space within us. In the absence of that emotional charge, there's more space inside to bring in positivity.

Picture a room with furniture in it. There's less room to bring in new stuff, but if you remove that furniture, there is more space for you to redecorate the room. What we're doing here with bringing in the positive stuff is redecorating the room now that there's more space in it. Let's bring in some positive stuff now that we've cleared out a lot of the more difficult stuff.

What Happens as We Clear the Trauma?

As we clear the emotional charge from the trauma, the nervous system can relax, and we're able to experience more joy, connection, love, and peace because the charge is no longer there. Trauma frequently impacts self-esteem and self-worth (Heller & LaPierre, 2012). When the charge is no longer there, these things will improve by themselves because the emotional weight that's been on us is no longer pulling us down. What we want to do then is bring in the positive beliefs and affirmation of who we are to support positive self-esteem.

How Do We Affirm Who We Are?

We can also use tapping to bring in positive beliefs after we clear the trauma. This occurs even while we are clearing the trauma by bringing love and acceptance to ourselves even while we're experiencing these difficult and complex emotions. Just by doing this, our sense of well-being and self-esteem improve. This is because we're telling ourselves, "I love you despite the fact that we're feeling that way. I accept you even while you're feeling this way."

We can do separate tapping processes that promote a greater sense of safety, trust, kindness, love, appreciation, and other qualities.

With trauma, we often forget who we are. We identify with the trauma, and the trauma can become part of our identity. It becomes who I am and how I define myself. If we look at the broader picture, trauma is only something that happened to you. It is not you. You are not your trauma. As we clear the charge, there's more space for us to notice that. Once we can shift that and no longer identify with the trauma, we can start to feel better. Clearing the trauma, cultivating self-knowledge, and learning about ourselves is how we establish a healthy identity.

In school, we learn a variety of skills. We learn about geography, math, science, and other subjects. What we almost universally don't learn about is ourselves. The more you know yourself and who you are, the more information you have. For example, knowing how you respond in certain situations and what your strengths are and are not, you can draw on your strengths more, and in doing so, you can feel better about yourself. The following three personality tests can be found online for free. They each give more information about who you are and how you conduct yourself in the world.

The VIA Character Strengths Survey tells you about your top five strengths (and all the others), which are very empowering (Peterson & Seligman, 2004). Let's say there's an issue that comes up in your life; you can ask yourself how you'd use your top five strengths to work through this issue.

Go to www.bit.ly/PTSDHealing to access the VIA strengths survey. Use Messenger keyword: strengths survey.

The Enneagram describes nine different personality types and what they look like in their underdeveloped, developed, and very developed stages (Riso & Hudson, 1999). Your Enneagram type can function as a road map for your own development. You get to see where you are now and what's possible for your personality type from this perspective. Select the classical test at the link below.

Go to www.bit.ly/PTSDHealing to access the Enneagram personality test. Use Messenger keyword: Enneagram.

Myers-Briggs is very similar. It shows how you work with the world and how you make decisions (Keirsey & Bates, 1998). Answer the questions at the link below with your first instinct. Don't overthink the questions.

Go to www.bit.ly/PTSDHealing to access the Myers-Briggs personality test. Use Messenger keyword: Myers-Briggs.

These tests are different lenses for looking at yourself. As you become familiar with yourself, you affirm your identity, and you become more comfortable with who you are. As a result, your self-esteem and self-worth improve naturally.

Self-Care

We bring in and sustain positivity through self-care. Self-care is any activity that restores well-being and brings you back to a space of alignment, relaxation, and openness. Culturally, in the US in particular, the prevalent norm seems to be overwork, lack of sleep, and productivity (Schulte, 2014). We seem to believe that overwork is what we should be striving for. We are judged based on how much we can produce and how much we can accomplish. The more we can accomplish, the better. When we accomplish less, we are evaluated more poorly. There's a focus on go, go, go, all the time, instead of rest time. The dominant question is about what was accomplished and what tangible outcomes I can physically point to as a result of that accomplishment.

These outcomes are best exhibited in the desire for the flashy car, fancy house, expensive phone, and so on. These things are prioritized over well-being. When we start to look at self-care, we are asserting that our own well-being is important. We get clear that we are willing to do the activities that are necessary and that feel good to ourselves, to cultivate, improve, and sustain our own well-being.

Self-Care Examples

Going for a walk	Adequate sleep
Taking an Epsom salt bath	Journaling
Yoga	Electronics-free time
Meditation	Gratitude journaling
Connecting with friends or romantic partners	Hiking
Alone time	Play
Eating nourishing food	Laughter
Time in nature	Time with your pet
Guided meditation	Listening to or playing music

Figure 10. Self-care examples.

Adults have almost universally lost the ability to play. Studies show that when you cultivate your ability to play, you're improving your creativity (Russ & Wallace, 2013). As adults, we're very clearly goal oriented. Play has no goal. There is no desired outcome with play. In that, there's less stress and more openness. In that openness, we can cultivate more creativity. Similarly, I think we have a tendency to take life too seriously, particularly in light of trauma. If we can cultivate more laughter, that too is medicine. All of these self-care activities are beneficial in their own ways.

Mindfulness

One of the items on the self-care list above is meditation. There's a myth that meditation is thinking about nothing. Somehow, you're supposed to sit there and focus on absolutely nothing.

From a mindfulness standpoint, meditation is using the breath or bodily sensations to be present in the moment. In other words, we're not wandering away in our mind. Mindfulness is essentially paying attention to what's here in the present moment with nonjudgment (Kabat-Zinn, 1991). We're noticing and acknowledging what's already here and practicing not judging it.

When we're triggered and we experience anger, we can think of that anger as the wound. From a Buddhist perspective, they call it the first arrow. If we judge the fact that we're angry, we're creating a second wound—the second arrow. If we notice when we have a judgment, we need to let go of it. It takes practice and attention to be able to notice judgments as they arise.

There's a quote by Carl Jung that roughly states, "What you resist persists." In other words, what you fight against you give negative energy to, which allows it to sustain itself or grow.

Let's use anger as an example. I notice that I'm angry and I start resisting that. If I tell myself I shouldn't feel angry, I am fighting against my current experience. That causes the situation to sustain itself.

Comparatively, if I can just notice it, like someone watching a movie, then I'm not fighting against it. I'm observing it with nonjudgmental awareness; that is mindfulness. That is also the foundational approach that we bring when we apply mindfulness meditation or when we use mindfulness throughout the day.

If you're eating food, you can engage your senses through your intentional awareness (David, 1991). You can pay attention to the tastes, the smells, and the sounds as you bite into it, the texture as you touch it, and hold it in your hands. You can incorporate all five of those senses into the experience of whatever you're doing now. You can be washing dishes and bring mindfulness to that. Mindfulness is something that you can bring to whatever it is that you're doing. It allows you to come back to the present moment by paying attention to your senses, your breath, or your bodily sensations. When you're paying attention to any of those things, you're not in the future thinking about what might happen, and you're also not in the past thinking about what happened because you're fully in the present, the now.

As you move into the mindfulness meditation exercise below, I want you to think about it like training a puppy (Harrington, 2013). When you train a puppy, you put out the little mat for it. It's supposed to pee on the mat. Instead, it'll wander away, and you have to gently bring the puppy back to the mat. It'll wander away again and you bring them back. Then it'll wander away again, and you bring it back again. This is your mind during meditation. There's some myth that great meditators are able to sit there and not have thoughts. You're going to have thoughts arise. The idea, then, is to gently and nonjudgmentally bring your attention back to your point of focus. If your breath is the focus of the meditation, bring your attention back to the breath.

You can record the exercise in your own voice by reading the meditation script below.
Go to www.bit.ly/PTSDHealing to access the mindfulness meditation exercise video and handout. Use Messenger keyword: mindfulness meditation.

Mindfulness Meditation Exercise

If it feels safe and comfortable to you, go ahead and close your eyes. If not, then just allow your eyes to relax and the lids to get heavy. Keep a barely open gaze toward the floor in front of you.

Find your breath here. Bring your attention to the sensation of the air coming in your nostrils and going out of your nostrils. Feel it coming in, going out, coming in, and going out. As you continue to breathe, bring your attention to the sensation of your chest rising as you inhale and coming back in as you exhale. Notice your belly expanding as you inhale and coming back in as you exhale. You can trace the path of the breath on an inhale from the nose all the way down to the belly. The belly expands as you inhale. As you exhale, the belly comes in, the breath comes up through the chest and out through the nose.

In through the nose and down through the chest and belly that expand. Then the breath comes up through the chest and out through the nose. Tracking the breath, noticing the breath, watching the breath. If paying attention to the belly and chest seems like too much right now, stay with the sensation of the breath coming in and out of the nose. Don't do anything to the breath to change it. Watch it as if you were watching a movie. In and out.

Notice where your attention is now. Bring it back to the breath.

Notice where you are now. Bring your attention back to your breath.

Now, gently begin to bring yourself back by noticing your bodily sensations. Notice where your body is touching your seat or contacting the floor. Take your time and at your own pace, gently open your eyes. Do you notice a difference in how you feel now compared to before that mindfulness practice?

We talked about short-term strategies for well-being, including self-care, internal awareness, clear communication, and cultivating a healthy sense of identity. We've also discussed long-term strategies for working with traumatic memories such as tapping, EMDR, cognitive processing, and exposure therapy.

Additional Thoughts about Self-Care

I have come to believe that caring for myself is not self-indulgent. Caring for myself is an act of survival.
—Audre Lorde

Self-care is giving the world what's best of you instead of what's left of you.

—Katie Reed

Almost everything will work again if you unplug it for a few minutes, including you.

—Anne Lamott

Self-care is so important. When you take time to replenish your spirit, it allows you to serve others from the overflow. You cannot serve from an empty vessel.

—Eleanor Brownn

If we don't take care of ourselves, we cannot show up the way we want to for ourselves and others.

Managing Daily Emotions

In a moment, you'll have an opportunity to practice one of my favorite processes for working with emotions. I use it all the time, and I recommend it to clients often. I call it the aura process. Earlier, we talked about the idea that what you resist persists. If you notice any difficult emotion like fear, shame, doubt, guilt, or sadness, you can use it. It can also be used with positive emotions like joy, peace, and love. When we talk about resistance for these purposes, generally we're talking about fighting against a more difficult emotion like I mentioned above. By fighting against them, they persist.

Culturally, emotional suppression is the norm. We're taught

to ignore our feelings, and we end up stuffing those emotions down. If we're feeling angry, we're saying to the anger, "I wish you weren't here," "leave me alone," or "go away." As a result, it remains. Since emotional suppression is the norm, we end up with a subconscious assumption that if we allow ourselves to actually feel our emotions, we're going to die. Somehow this emotion will be so strong that it will overwhelm and kill us. The truth is, if we give these emotions the room that they need to breathe and integrate, they usually move through.

To say that a little differently, when we fight against them, they stay and hang out. When we actually give them the space they need to breathe, they move through. With this process we're going in the opposite direction, we are not resisting. On one end of a spectrum, we're fighting against them, pushing them down, and wishing they weren't here. With this process we're going to the end of the spectrum by saying, "Hey, I see you, anger, and it's okay for you to be here right now. You know what? I'm going to give you all the space I possibly can so that you integrate and move through." Rumi beautifully captures this welcoming sentiment as translated by Coleman Barks (1996):

The Guest House

This being human is a guest house.
Every morning a new arrival.

A joy, a depression, a meanness,
some momentary awareness comes
as an unexpected visitor.

> Welcome and entertain them all!
> Even if they are a crowd of sorrows,
> who violently sweep your house
> empty of its furniture,
> still, treat each guest honorably.
> He may be clearing you out
> for some new delight.
>
> The dark thought, the shame, the malice.
> Meet them at the door laughing and invite them in.
>
> Be grateful for whatever comes.
> Because each has been sent
> as a guide from beyond.

Many of the themes that we've been discussing are echoed in this poem. Using mindfulness to notice our feelings and welcome those feelings nonjudgmentally, regardless of what they are, goes against the cultural norm, but it's so healthy for us. We're using those feelings as a guide from beyond as we notice what's here. This process that you're about to do is how I welcome these guests into the guest house. I am the guest house. You are the guest house. Now, we'll see how we can welcome these feelings and give them the space they need.

Aura Process Practice

If it feels safe and comfortable, go ahead and close your eyes. If not, allow your eyes to relax and the lids to get heavy. Keep a barely open gaze toward the floor in front of you.

Go to www.bit.ly/PTSDHealing to access the aura process video and handout. Use Messenger keyword: aura process.

For this exercise, notice what emotion you are feeling now before we begin.

1. Ask yourself, "What emotion am I feeling?" Name the emotion. "I am feeling _____."

    It might be that "I'm feeling relaxed." "I'm feeling joy." "I'm feeling sad." "I'm feeling relief." "I'm feeling raw." "I'm feeling vulnerable." Whatever the emotion is, make sure you use an emotion word. *Good* and *bad* are far too vague.

2. Ask yourself, "Where do I feel this emotion in my body?" Notice the location in your body. Notice the quality of the sensation. What does the sensation feel like in your body?

    You might feel it in your belly, chest, head, or your big toe. The sensation might be pulsing, tight, heavy, light, or tingly.

3. Take a long inhale and visualize expanding this emotion through your whole body. Long exhale.

    This may seem counterintuitive or counterproductive, but try it anyway.

4. Take a long inhale and visualize expanding this emotion through your body and your aura. Exhale.

    Go three feet out on all sides of you: three feet to your left, right, in front, in back, above, and below.

5. Take a long inhale and visualize, creating an ocean of this feeling behind you.

6. Exhale and allow yourself to fall back into the ocean of this feeling. You can invite in someone to support you in falling in if that feels helpful.

Breathe here. Notice what you're experiencing now. What is your emotional experience now compared to before you did this process?

If you're by yourself and have some difficult feelings come up, you can use this process. If you're interacting with someone and you have some difficult feelings come up, you can do this process. If you're in the middle of a crowded room, you can apply this process.

This is what I call a rinse-and-repeat process. I'll do this myself and with clients. The emotion will integrate after one repetition—one cycle of these six steps. Generally, if the emotion doesn't integrate after one repetition, it will integrate after two repetitions. For extremely triggering stuff, it may take you five or more repetitions to create space internally. It also allows us to come back to alignment with our true selves. It gives us more choice in how we respond because we're taking the time to integrate and work with what's happening with us instead of reacting to whatever is happening outside us immediately. It allows us to come back to the present moment where we have a lot more opportunity to find peace and well-being since we're not anxiously thinking about the future or depressed thinking about the past.

Violet Flame Practice Process

This next process can be used by itself or after the aura process. It shouldn't be used to bypass how you're feeling, but it can help break up and release heavy, dense, or stagnant energy.

Feel free to record a version yourself.

Go to www.bit.ly/PTSDHealing to access the violet flame process video and handout. Use Messenger keyword: violet flame.

Go ahead and close your eyes. If you want to keep them cracked, that's perfectly fine too as long as your gaze is relaxed. For those of us that are comfortable, I want to encourage you to close your eyes.

Focus on your breath again. Keep your attention on it as it goes in and out, in and out.

Visualize now that your entire body is surrounded by a violet flame. This flame is totally safe and comfortable.

Continue to breathe as you inhale see this violet flame entering into every cell of your body. Every cell of your body is glowing with the violet flame so strongly that if you opened your eyes right now and looked in a mirror, you would see it glowing through your skin. This violet flame breaks down all negative energy within your body at the particle level. The violet flame extracts all these particles of negative energy through your skin, and they collect in a cloud outside of you. You might see them shift from the purple color into a golden color or whatever color feels right to you as they become positive, supportive energy.

See that positive, supportive energy fall away down past your feet, down through the floor, down into the soil beneath the floor, and where it nourishes the soil and the earth.

Visualize now that your entire body and your aura are surrounded by the violet flame, going three feet out on all sides of you: to your left, right, in front, behind, above, and below.

The violet flame breaks down all negative energy within your entire body and your aura at the particle level. The violet flame extracts all these particles of negative energy through your skin, and they collect in a cloud outside of you.

These particles that are now in the air outside of you are still glowing with the violet flame. The violet flame transforms those particles into positive, supportive energy. You might see them shift from the purple color into a golden color or whatever color feels right to you as they become positive, supportive energy.

See that positive, supportive energy fall away down past your feet, down through the floor, down into the soil beneath the floor, and where it nourishes the soil and the earth.

Visualize now that your entire body, your aura, and your field are surrounded by the violet flame, going 25 feet out on all sides of you: to your left, right, in front, behind, above, and below.

The violet flame breaks down all negative energy within your entire body, your aura, and your field at the particle level. The violet flame extracts all these particles of negative energy through your skin, and they collect in a cloud outside of you.

The violet flame transforms those particles into positive, supportive energy. You might see them shift from the purple color into a golden color or whatever color feels right to you as they become positive, supportive energy.

See that positive, supportive energy fall away down past your feet, down through the floor, down into the soil beneath the floor, and where it nourishes the soil and the earth.

Breathing here, notice how you feel now compared to before that process. You just did energy work at home! Taking your time, breathe normally, and open your eyes when you're ready.

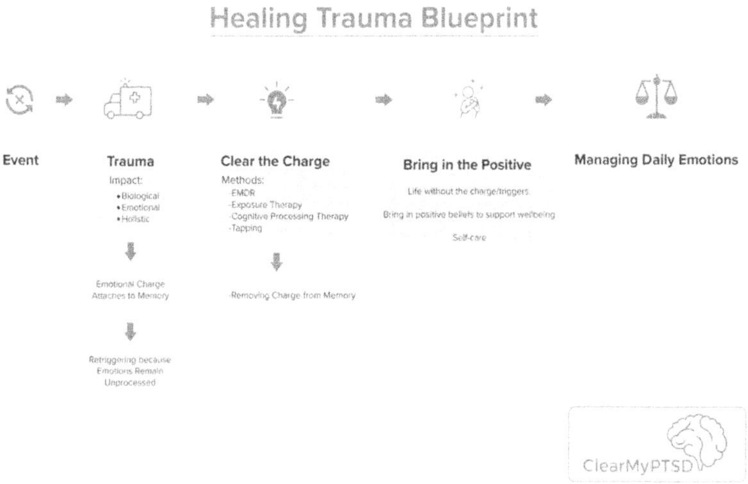

Healing Trauma Blueprint

Figure 11. The healing trauma blueprint.

In this chapter, we've talked about the event and the emotional charge that we experience around the event that leads to trauma (figure 11). We've talked about the importance of doing the deeper work to clear the charge. I recommended tapping as a go-to method for that. As we clear the charge, we see that there's more space inside and we're able to bring in more positive energy and beliefs to start feeling even better. We also understand how clearing the charge and bringing in more positivity leads to improved self-esteem and self-worth. We've talked about incorporating more self-care and managing emotions daily and using the aura process and the violet flame specifically as a means of doing that.

What It Really Looks Like

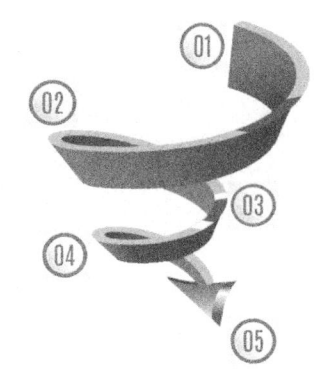

1. The event

2. Trauma

    Biological, holistic, and emotional perspectives

    a. Adverse childhood experiences (ACEs)

3. Clearing the charge

    EMDR, exposure therapy, cognitive reprocessing therapy, and tapping

    a. Tapping process overview

4. **Bringing in the Positive**

   Life without the charge; self-care

   a. Meditation exercise

5. **Managing daily emotions**

   Working with emotions day to day

   a. Aura process exercise

   b. Violet flame

Above is the healing trauma blueprint we looked at earlier (figure 11). The second image is what the healing trauma process really looks like (figure 12). The diagram is a spiral. We go deeper and deeper. First, we have an event, and then we have the trauma in response to the event. Then we clear the charge from the trauma. In doing so, we're able to have more space inside to bring in positive beliefs. Then, we manage our emotions from day to day and moment to moment. For a lot of folks, there are multiple traumas, so we go through this process multiple times. Each time we go deeper.

To say that a little differently, we are clearing the charge from multiple traumas. Just like your house, if you clear out the furniture from one room and then a second room, there is even more space in the house to bring in new furniture and to redecorate. The more trauma and wounds there are and the more emotional charge that we can clear out, the more space we have to bring in positive energy, positive beliefs, and improved well-being. I want to offer a word of caution here. In our culture, there's a tendency to push and be hard on ourselves. That same approach can unconsciously be applied to the healing process as well. We can be unkind and mean to ourselves while we're trying to heal. You may think you should have healed a particular thing by now, make faster progress, or that you should be doing better than you are. Instead, intentionally go at your own pace—a pace that's right for you. Be kind to yourself.

Einstein said, "If you always do what you always did, you will always get what you always got." He also said, "Insanity is doing the same thing over and over again and expecting different results." Practice when it feels good and at the same time balance that out with not putting it off either. It's finding the balance between not pressuring yourself, not being hard on yourself or unkind to yourself but also doing what you need to do to pursue your own healing and to come back to a space of well-being.

In closing, Rumi said, "The wound is the place where the Light enters you." The more you clear out the trauma and wounding that keeps you from embodying your true self, the more light that can shine through you.

Go to www.bit.ly/PTSDHealing to access the full cheat sheet and chapter summary. Use Messenger keyword: chapter one cheat sheet.

Chapter One Brief Summary

- Trauma results from an emotional charge in response to an event that our system cannot tolerate.
- From the holistic, biological and emotional perspectives, trauma is stuck energy.

- Integrating the stuck energy (emotional charge) can be done many ways; I am recommending Tapping as it is the most effective according to research studies.

- Once we clear the emotional charge we can bring in positive beliefs with Tapping.

- Beyond healing the trauma, managing daily emotions is also an essential part of the process and can similarly be done with Tapping.

To delve deeper into the core components of trauma and Tapping, and to receive step by step instructions to drastically reduce your PTSD, join us for the Clear My PTSD Healing Accelerator at www.ClearMyPTSD.com/course

CHAPTER 2:

CONQUERING THE SADNESS, ANXIETY, DEPRESSION, ANGER, FEAR, AND OVERWHELM—HOW TO USE TAPPING TO MANAGE DAILY EMOTIONS

In This Chapter

In this chapter, we're going to cover a tapping overview, walk through the tapping points, and then practice them. Then we'll practice them again with my two favorite techniques: breath and sound followed by a sample tapping process. After that, we'll look at how to incorporate tapping daily.

Tapping Overview

Let's look again at an overview of tapping. Tapping is based on the idea that we have life force energy which flows through small energy centers called meridians. Meridians are like power lines that flow through our system, bringing the energy where it needs to go (Solomon, 2007). These meridians are responsible for our emotions and our organs. From an Eastern medicine perspective, all disease—physical, mental, emotional, or spiritual—is caused by a block in the flow of energy. What we're doing with tapping is restoring the flow of energy through the system. The system has its own wisdom and restores itself in the absence of blocks.

Here is the complete tapping process (Church, 2013):

Complete tapping process
1. Measure the emotion before (0-10).
2. Make an opening statement.
3. Start tapping sequence part one with sighs.
4. Do The 9-Gamut Procedure.
5. Do tapping sequence part two with sighs.
6. Measure the emotion afterward (0-10).

This may look like a lot, and it might even look strange as we begin. By the end, this will all make sense. To give an overview: Prior to beginning a round of tapping, we want to measure the intensity of what's going on from 0 to 10. We then make an opening statement that tells our subconscious what it is we're working on. We then go through a tapping sequence where we tap through the points. Next, we do what I call the intermission process, which is the 9-Gamut Procedure (Craig & Fowlie, 1995). We tap on a particular point and do a whole bunch of things while we're tapping there. Following that, we tap through the points again, and then measure again from 0 to

10. We measure from 0 to 10 before *and* after a tapping round. For example, if we start a tapping round with an intensity of 8, we might measure at the end of the round and find that we're at a 6. We can go through and do another tapping round and find ourselves at a 2 intensity. We can see to what extent we've made progress by virtue of measuring before and afterward.

If the tapping instructions below seem confusing or overwhelming, don't worry. They will be covered shortly in more detail below with video guidance available as well. You don't have to memorize this information. It's just to get a sense of what the process looks like.

These are the tapping points for the first half of a tapping round (Church, 2013):

Tapping sequence part one	
1. L. karate chop	10. Solar plexus
2. Eyebrow	11. Left wrist
3. Side of the eye	12. Side of l. thumb
4. Cheekbone	13. Side of l. index
5. Upper lip	14. Side of l. middle
6. Lower lip	15. Underside l. ring
7. Collarbone	16. Underside l. pinky
8. Heart	17. L. karate chop
9. Armpit	

Bilateral Stimulation in Tapping

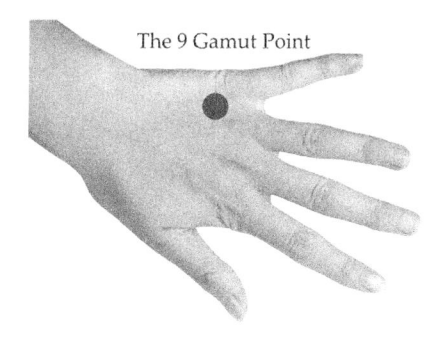

Figure 12: The 9-gamut point.

Intermission: The 9-Gamut Procedure
1. Continuously tap on this point.
2. Look down to the left.
3. Look down to the right.
4. Roll the eyes to the left in a full circle.
5. Roll the eyes to the right in a full circle.
6. Count to five.
7. Hum a tune for a few seconds.
8. Count to seven.
9. Hum a tune for a few seconds.

Then we have the intermission process (Church, 2013). For the intermission process, there's only one point (figure 12). It's located on your hand between the knuckles of the pinky and ring finger. While we're tapping on that point, we do a whole bunch of funny-looking things. The goal of doing these things is to activate and align both hemispheres of our brain. This brings the whole brain online to process whatever it is that we're working through in this round of tapping. As a result, we have more integration. We saw earlier that when we experience trauma, there is stuck energy in our energy system. When we bring more of our brain online to process it, the stuck energy can move through our system more easily. We're bringing more of our resources to the table where maybe those resources weren't present when we initially encountered whatever caused the issue.

These are the tapping points for the second half of a tapping round (Church, 2013):

Tapping sequence part two	
1. Eyebrow	9. Solar plexus
2. Side of the eye	10. Right wrist
3. Cheekbone	11. Side of r. thumb
4. Upper lip	12. Side of r. index
5. Lower lip	13. Side of r. middle
6. Collarbone	14. Underside r. ring
7. Heart	15. Underside r. pinky
8. Armpit	16. R. karate chop

The second half of a tapping round is very similar to the first half (Church, 2013). There are two main differences. We're not starting with the karate chop point, and we're tapping on the right side of the body.

Tapping Sequence Part One

We can see that when we do part one of the round, we're starting with the left karate chop point and we're going through the left-hand points. So the idea is first, we do the left side of the body, go through the intermission process, and then we do the right side of the body. We tap on each point about seven times, though there is no need to count. All of these meridian points correspond to different organs and emotions. By tapping on these points, we're stimulating the flow of energy in our system, signaling it to wake up.

Below is a practice process to get familiar with the tapping points.

Go to www.bit.ly/PTSDHealing to access the tapping points introduction video and handout. Use Messenger keyword: tapping points introduction.

Practicing the Tapping Points

Before we begin, take stock of how you're feeling now. Notice what emotions are present now. Take the lay of the land and see what's here now before we go through this process. We are getting a feel for the tapping points, and we're just noticing how we feel before we do that. Then we'll see how we feel after we go through this process. Once you have a sense of how you're feeling, continue through the points below.

Make sure you're not tapping so softly that you can't feel it. Make sure you're not being unkind to yourself by tapping too hard.

1. **Left karate chop.** Take your left hand and extend it in a karate chop as if you're about to chop wood. Take the four fingertips of the right hand and bring them to the karate chop area of the left hand. Make sure you're tapping on the meaty portion of the hand with your fingertips.

2. **Eyebrow.** Bring the two index and the middle fingertips of both hands to the furry part of the eyebrows, right where they meet the nose. Tap there for a few moments.

3. **Side of the eye.** Tap on the temples, which are outside the eyebrows. You can feel there's a small indentation in the skull. Tap there.

4. **Cheekbone.** Tap on the cheekbones directly below the eyes. Your fingers should be directly in line with your eyes.

5. **Upper lip.** With the fingertips of the index and middle fingers of one hand, tap below the nose in the crevice in the upper lip.

6. **Lower lip.** Now tap in the crevice above the chin and below the bottom lip.

7. **Collarbone.** Now we're going to find the collarbone point. To me, this is the most difficult point to find. Feel your collarbones at the top of your chest. Below your collarbones is a hollow area. You can feel the sternum there as well, running up and down. Using your dominant hand, place your thumb on one side of it and your index and middle finger on the other side. You'll know it's the right place because it's soft there. Make sure that your thumb, index,

and middle fingers are as close to your sternum as possible. Tap there for a moment.

8. **Heart.** Place all four fingertips of your tapping hand right on your sternum above the heart. Tap there.

9. **Armpit.** Now tap on the armpit points. This is going to be four inches below your armpits. Tap around in this area and see if there are any tender spots. If there are tender spots, tap right on them. If not, tap four inches below your armpits.

10. **Solar plexus.** Find your solar plexus at the base of the ribs. Tap from the center of your bottom ribs out along the bottom ribs toward your sides. See if you can find any tender spots there. If you find any tender spots, tap right on them. If not, you can tap directly in line with the nipples.

11. **Left wrist.** Extend your left hand palm up toward the sky. Take the two fingertips of your right hand and tap on the center of the left wrist right where it meets the hand.

12. **Side of the left thumb.** Then tap on the side of the left thumb, right by the nail, not on the nail or the underside of the finger. If you were to try to chop a piece of wood, this would be the part of your thumb that is facing toward the ceiling.

Make sure you're using your fingertips to tap directly on each point.

13. **Side of the left index finger.** Tap on the side of the index finger on the same spot. Tap right on the side where the nail is but not on the nail.

14. **Side of the left middle finger.** Do the same with the middle finger.

    Keep your left hand still and just move your right hand. Leave the tapping fingers of the right hand extended as you rotate the tapping hand palm up toward the ceiling.

15. **Underside of the left ring finger.** Bring the fingertips onto the underside of your ring finger by the nail. If you were chopping wood with your left hand, it would be the side of your ring finger facing the ground.

16. **Underside of the left pinky finger.** Continue tapping on the same spot on the pinky finger.

17. **Left karate chop.** Bring all four of your right fingertips back to the meaty portion of your left hand. Tap right on the meaty portion.

    Shake out your tapping hands. That was half a round of tapping. Check in now and notice how you're feeling compared to before.

The Two Secret Techniques: Breath and Sound

In yoga, breath is translated as pranayama. Pranayama means breathwork practice, life force, and energy control. When we inhale, even when we're breathing normally, we are bringing in new energy. When we exhale, we're casting out old energy. Any time we lengthen our inhale, we're increasing the amount of new energy we're bringing in. Any time we lengthen our exhale we're increasing the amount of old energy we're casting out and letting go.

Sound is a particularly potent healing element. In India, mantras have been chanted for thousands of years. In the US, sound is being used to do things like breaking up kidney stones so that they can be released. When we invoke sound, we can align ourselves with different frequencies that have different healing benefits. I find a lot of folks hold back and repress themselves, refraining from expressing what they really want to say. If we can give ourselves permission to let the sound out through the tapping process, we're releasing that much more.

Using the process below, we'll practice incorporating the breath (Hartmann, 2003) and sound (Singh, 2015) into the tapping process by sighing after we tap on each point.

Go to www.bit.ly/PTSDHealing to access the tapping with breath and sound video and handout. Use Messenger keyword: breath and sound.

Practicing the Tapping Points with Sound and Breath

Before we begin, take stock of how you're feeling now. Notice what emotions are present now. Take the lay of the land and see what's here now before we go through this process. We are about to get a feel for tapping through the points with sound and breath, and we're just noticing how we feel before we do that. Then we'll see how we feel after we do that.

1. **Right karate chop: deep inhale, sigh. (Repeat with sigh three times.)** Take your right hand and extend it in a karate chop as if you're about to chop wood. Take the four fingertips of the left hand and bring them to the karate chop area of the right hand. Make sure you're tapping on the meaty portion of the hand with your fingertips.

2. **Eyebrow: deep inhale, sigh.** Bring the two index and the middle fingertips of both hands to the furry part of the eyebrows, right where they meet the nose. Tap there for a few moments.

3. **Side of the eye: deep inhale, sigh.** Then tap on the temples, which are outside the eyebrows. You can feel there's a small indentation in the skull. Tap there.

4. **Cheekbone: deep inhale, sigh.** Tap on the cheekbones directly below the eyes. Your fingers should be directly in line with your eyes.

5. **Upper lip: deep inhale, sigh.** With the fingertips of the index and middle fingers of one hand, tap below the nose in the crevice in the upper lip.

6. **Lower lip: deep inhale, sigh.** Now tap in the crevice above the chin and below the bottom lip.

7. **Collarbone: deep inhale, sigh.** Now we're going to find the collarbone point. To me, this is the most difficult point to find. Feel your collarbones at the top of your chest. Below your collarbones is a hollow area. You can feel the sternum there as well, running up and down. Using your

dominant hand, place your thumb on one side of it and your index and middle finger on the other side. You'll know it's the right spot because it's soft there. Make sure that your thumb, index, and middle fingers are as close to your sternum as possible. Tap there for a moment.

8. **Heart: deep inhale, sigh.** Place all four fingertips of your tapping hand right on your sternum above the heart. Tap there.

9. **Armpit: deep inhale, sigh.** Now tap on the armpit points. This is four inches below your armpits. Tap around in this area and see if you can find any tender spots. If there are tender spots, tap right on them. If not, tap four inches below your armpits.

10. **Solar plexus: deep inhale, sigh.** Find your solar plexus at the base of the ribs. Tap from the center of your bottom ribs out along the bottom ribs toward your sides. Notice any tender spots there. If you find any tender spots, tap right on them. If not, you can tap directly in line with the nipples.

11. **Right wrist: deep inhale, sigh.** Extend your right hand palm up toward the sky. Take the two fingertips of your left hand and tap on the center of the right wrist right where it meets the hand.

12. **Side of the right thumb: deep inhale, sigh.** Then tap on the side of the right thumb by the nail, not on the nail or the underside of the finger. If you were to try to chop a

piece of wood, this would be the part of your thumb that is facing toward the ceiling.

Make sure you're using your fingertips to tap directly on each point.

13. **Side of the right index finger: deep inhale, sigh.** Tap on the side of the index finger on the same spot. Tap on the side where the nail is but not on the nail.

14. **Side of the right middle finger: deep inhale, sigh.** Repeat with the middle finger.

    Keep your right hand still and just move your left hand. Leave the tapping fingers of the left hand extended as you rotate the tapping hand palm up toward the ceiling.

15. **Underside of the right ring finger: deep inhale, sigh.** Bring the fingertips onto the underside of your ring finger by the nail. If you were chopping wood with your right hand, it would be the side of your ring finger facing the ground.

16. **Underside of the right pinky finger: deep inhale, sigh.** Continue tapping the same spot on the pinky finger.

17. **Right karate chop: deep inhale, sigh.** Bring all four of your fingertips to the meaty portion of your right hand. Tap right on the meaty portion. Take a nice deep inhale. Give yourself permission to make the biggest sigh you've done all day. Repeat that huge inhale and sigh a second time.

Shake out your tapping hands. That was half a round of tapping. Check in now and notice how you're feeling compared to before going through this process with sound and breath.

Two Types of Tapping: Additive and Reductive

I divide tapping into two types: additive and reductive. Broadly speaking, reductive tapping is where we're releasing and integrating what's already here. Additive tapping is when we're bringing in what we want more of. Essentially, we're adding and subtracting—adding and reducing.

Exploring the Two Types of Tapping

Reductive tapping (Ortner, 2014) is where you integrate and release a difficult experience. We do that by bringing love and acceptance to what's already here.

Additive tapping (Dawson & Marillat, 2014) is where you are bringing in the positive, your true wants, and desires. As a general rule, I encourage people to do reductive tapping first. That way we're clearing out and integrating the difficult experience before we bring in what we want. Going back to the metaphor for redecorating your home, this is where we're cleaning out the rooms first so that we can redecorate during the additive portion.

Preparation for a Reductive Tapping Process

Shortly, you'll practice a reductive tapping process. First, we're going to do some preparation for that. As we discussed in the beginning of the first chapter, Rumi said, "Your task is not to seek love but merely to seek and find all the barriers you have built against it." With this process, we're clearing out those barriers.

Notice how you feel now. Take stock of what's here. This is a mindfulness exercise where we're just bringing awareness and attention to how we're doing inside.

Once you have the flavor of that, think about the most difficult memory from this past week—the most difficult situation.

When you have that memory, notice what the most difficult and dominant emotion related to it is.

To help with this, you can use the feelings inventory from the Center for Nonviolent Communication with the link below. On it, you'll see feelings when your needs are being met and feelings when your needs are not being met (Rosenberg, 2003). Feelings when your needs are being met might include joy, contentment, peace, etc. Feelings when your needs are not being met might include anger, sadness, fear, etc. This inventory can help you find a word to describe the most difficult emotion from that experience. There are different feeling categories. Under each category, there are nuanced flavors for that feeling. Name the feeling when you have it.

Go to www.bit.ly/PTSDHealing to access the feelings inventory. Use Messenger keyword: feelings inventory.

For this practice process, we'll use the feeling of being depressed. However, feel free to plug in whatever your dominant feeling is every time I use the word depressed.

Visualize the memory for a moment so you can get a feel for the intensity of that *depressed* feeling from 0 to 10. Write that number down.

Making an opening statement
1. Even though I am feeling_____ [difficult emotion], I deeply and profoundly love and accept myself.
a. Examples:
i. Even though <u>I am feeling this anger</u>, I deeply and profoundly love and accept myself.
ii. Even though <u>I am feeling this sadness</u>, I deeply and profoundly love and accept myself.
2. Repeat the opening statement three times while tapping on the left karate chop point at the beginning of a tapping round.
3. Be as specific as possible.

Now we'll make an opening statement. This is something that we do at the beginning of a reductive tapping round, typically. Below, what we have is a formula. The formula follows a pattern of "Even though [whatever the issue is], I deeply and profoundly love and accept myself."

In this example we'd say, "Even though I'm feeling this <u>depression</u>, I deeply and profoundly love and accept myself." Then we would repeat the opening statement three times while tapping on the karate chop point at the beginning of a tapping round. We want to be as specific as possible about what it is that we're tapping on. Now you have an opening statement.

Next, we'll create a reminder phrase.

Creating a reminder phrase
1. A short phrase used while tapping on each point in the sequence
a. Example:
i. **Opening statement:** Even though <u>I am feeling this sadness</u>, I deeply and profoundly love and accept myself.
ii. **Reminder phrase:** <u>this sadness</u>
b. Example:
i. **Opening statement:** Even though <u>I am feeling this anger toward my father</u>, I deeply and profoundly love and accept myself.
ii. **Reminder phrase:** <u>this anger</u>

The reminder phrase is a very short phrase that we use while we're tapping on each point as we go through the round. In other words, after we do the opening statement three times, this is the phrase we'll be using on each point as we go through the remainder of the round.

In this example, as we've said, the opening statement would be "Even though I'm feeling this <u>depression</u>, I deeply and profoundly love and accept myself." The reminder phrase would be "<u>this depression</u>."

We have identified the intensity of the feeling in the memory and created an opening statement as well as a reminder phrase to work with it. Now we'll go through a whole reductive tapping practice round. After the tapping round, we'll measure the intensity again.

Go to www.bit.ly/PTSDHealing to access the reductive tapping practice round video and handout. Use Messenger keyword: full practice round.

The First Half of the Reductive Tapping Practice Round

1. **Left karate chop.** Say aloud, "Even though I'm feeling this <u>depression</u>, I deeply and profoundly love and accept myself." Repeat three times, followed by a **deep inhale and a sigh**.

   Take your left hand and extend it in a karate chop as if you're about to chop wood. Take the four fingertips of the right hand and bring them to the karate chop area of the left hand. Make sure you're tapping on the meaty portion of the hand with your fingertips.

2. **Eyebrow.** Say aloud, "This depression," followed by a **deep inhale and a sigh**.

   Bring the two index and the middle fingertips of both hands to the furry part of the eyebrows, right where they meet the nose. Tap there for a few moments.

3. **Side of the eye.** Say aloud, "This depression," followed by a **deep inhale and a sigh**.

   Then tap on the temples, which are outside the eyebrows. You can feel there's a small indentation in the skull. Tap there.

4. **Cheekbone.** Say aloud, "This depression," followed by a **deep inhale and a sigh**.

   Tap on the cheekbones directly below the eyes. Your fingers should be directly in line with your eyes.

5. **Upper lip.** Say aloud, "This depression," followed by a **deep inhale and a sigh.**

   With the fingertips of the index and middle fingers of one hand, tap below the nose in the crevice in the upper lip.

6. **Lower lip.** Say aloud, "This depression," followed by a **deep inhale and a sigh.**

   Now tap in the crevice above the chin and below the bottom lip.

7. **Collarbone.** Say aloud, "This depression," followed by a **deep inhale and a sigh.**

   Now we're going to find the collarbone point. To me, this is the most difficult point to find. Feel your collarbones at the top of your chest. Below your collarbones is a hollow area. You can feel the sternum there as well, running up and down. Using your dominant hand, place your thumb on one side of it and your index and middle finger on the other side. You'll know it's the right place because it's soft there. Make sure that your thumb, index, and middle fingers are as close to your sternum as possible. Tap there for a moment.

8. **Heart.** Say aloud, "This depression," followed by a **deep inhale and a sigh.**

   Place all four fingertips of your tapping hand right on your sternum above the heart. Tap there.

9. **Armpit.** Say aloud, "This depression," followed by a **deep inhale and a sigh.**

Now tap on the armpit points. This is four inches below your armpits. Tap around in this area and see if there are any tender spots. If there are tender spots, tap right on them. If not, tap four inches below your armpits.

10. **Solar plexus.** Say aloud, "This depression," followed by a **deep inhale and a sigh**.

    Find your solar plexus at the base of the ribs. Tap from the center of your bottom ribs out along the bottom ribs toward your sides. See if you can find any tender spots there. If you find any tender spots, tap right on them. If not, you can tap directly in line with the nipples.

11. **Left wrist.** Say aloud, "This depression," followed by a **deep inhale and a sigh**.

    Extend your left hand palm up toward the sky. Take the two fingertips of your right hand and tap on the center of the left wrist right where it meets the hand.

12. **Side of the left thumb.** Say aloud, "This depression," followed by a **deep inhale and a sigh**.

    Then tap on the side of the left thumb, right by the nail, not on the nail or the underside of the finger. If you were to try to chop a piece of wood, this would be the part of your thumb that is facing toward the ceiling.

    Make sure you're using your fingertips to tap directly on each point.

13. **Side of the left index finger.** Say aloud, "This depression," followed by a **deep inhale and a sigh**.

Tap on the side of the index finger on the same spot. Tap right on the side where the nail is but not on the nail.

14. **Side of the left middle finger.** Say aloud, "This depression," followed by a **deep inhale and a sigh.**

    Do the same with the middle finger.

    Keep your left hand still and just move your right hand. Leave the tapping fingers of the right hand extended as you rotate the tapping hand palm up toward the ceiling.

15. **Underside of the left ring finger.** Say aloud, "This depression," followed by a **deep inhale and a sigh.**

    Bring the fingertips onto the underside of your ring finger by the nail. If you were chopping wood with your left hand, it would be the side of your ring finger facing the ground.

16. **Underside of the left pinky finger.** Say aloud, "This depression," followed by a **deep inhale and a sigh.**

    Continue tapping on the same spot on the pinky finger.

17. **Left karate chop.** Say aloud, "This depression," followed by a **deep inhale and a sigh.**

    Bring all four of your fingertips back to the meaty portion of the left hand. Tap right on the meaty portion.

Now we're going to do the intermission process by tapping on the 9-gamut point (Craig & Fowlie, 1995).

Practicing the 9-Gamut Procedure

Take the two fingertips of your right hand and find the knuckles of your left ring finger and pinky finger. Place your two fingertips there. Trace your fingertips back toward the wrist about an inch higher than the knuckles (figure 12). You'll find a hollow area there. Place the fingertips of your index and middle fingers there. Tap here for the remainder of the 9-Gamut Procedure (Craig & Fowlie, 1995).

1. Keep your chin parallel to the floor. Do not move your head throughout this process. Continue to tap on this point.
2. Keeping your head still, look down to the left.
3. Look down to the right.
4. Roll your eyes completely to the right.
5. Roll your eyes completely to the left.
6. Count to five out loud.
7. Hum a tune for a few seconds.

    I like to use "Oh, when the saints." Use a real tune instead of making one up.

8. Count to seven out loud.
9. Hum a tune again.

We've done the first half of a tapping round followed by the intermission process. If this were a sandwich, that would be one piece of bread followed by the filling for the sandwich, and now we're going to add in the second piece of bread to complete the sandwich by doing the second half.

The Second Half of the Reductive Practice Round

1. **Eyebrow.** Say aloud, "This depression," followed by a **deep inhale and a sigh.**

   Bring the two index and the middle fingertips of both hands to the furry part of the eyebrows, right where they meet the nose. Tap there for a few moments.

2. **Side of the eye.** Say aloud, "This depression," followed by a **deep inhale and a sigh.**

   Then tap on the temples, which are outside the eyebrows. You can feel there's a small indentation in the skull there. Tap there.

3. **Cheekbone.** Say aloud, "This depression," followed by a **deep inhale and a sigh.**

   Tap on the cheekbones directly below the eyes. Your fingers should be directly in line with your eyes.

4. **Upper lip.** Say aloud, "This depression," followed by a **deep inhale and a sigh.**

   With the fingertips of the index and middle fingers of one hand, tap below the nose in the crevice in the upper lip.

5. **Lower lip.** Say aloud, "This depression," followed by a **deep inhale and a sigh.**

Now tap in the crevice above the chin and below the bottom lip.

6. **Collarbone.** Say aloud, "This depression," followed by a **deep inhale and a sigh**.

   Now we're going to find the collarbone point. To me, this is the most difficult point to find. Feel your collarbones at the top of your chest. Below your collarbones is a hollow area. You can feel the sternum there as well, running up and down. Using your dominant hand, place your thumb on one side of it and your index and middle finger on the other side. You'll know it's the right spot because it's soft there. Make sure that your thumb, index, and middle fingers are as close to your sternum as possible. Tap there for a moment.

7. **Heart.** Say aloud, "This depression," followed by a **deep inhale and a sigh**.

   Place all four fingertips of your tapping hand right on your sternum above the heart. Tap there.

8. **Armpit.** Say aloud, "This depression," followed by a **deep inhale and a sigh**.

   Now tap on the armpit points. This is four inches below your armpits. Tap around in this area and see if there are any tender spots. If there are tender spots, tap right on them. If not, tap four inches below your armpits.

9. **Solar plexus.** Say aloud, "This depression," followed by a **deep inhale and a sigh**.

Find your solar plexus at the base of the ribs. Tap from the center of your bottom ribs out along the bottom ribs toward your sides. See if you can find any tender spots there. If you find any tender spots, tap right on them. If not, you can tap directly in line with the nipples.

10. **Right wrist.** Say aloud, "This depression," followed by a **deep inhale and a sigh.**

    Extend your right hand palm up toward the sky. Take the two fingertips of your left hand and tap on the center of the right wrist right where it meets the hand.

11. **Side of the right thumb.** Say aloud, "This depression," followed by a **deep inhale and a sigh.**

    Then tap on the side of the right thumb by the nail, not on the nail or the underside of the finger. If you were to try to chop a piece of wood, this would be the part of your thumb that is facing toward the ceiling.

    Make sure you're using your fingertips to tap directly on each point.

12. **Side of the right index finger.** Say aloud, "This depression," followed by a **deep inhale and a sigh.**

    Tap on the side of the index finger on the same spot. Tap on the side where the nail is but not on the nail.

13. **Side of the right middle finger.** Say aloud, "This depression," followed by a **deep inhale and a sigh.**

    Do the same with the middle finger.

Then, keep your right hand still and just move your left hand. Leave the tapping fingers of the left hand extended as you rotate the tapping hand palm up toward the ceiling.

14. **Underside of the right ring finger.** Say aloud, "This depression," followed by a **deep inhale and a sigh**.

    Bring the fingertips onto the underside of your ring finger by the nail. If you were chopping wood with your right hand, it would be the side of your ring finger facing the ground.

15. **Underside of the right pinky finger.** Say aloud, "This depression," followed by a **deep inhale and a sigh**.

    Continue tapping the same spot on the pinky finger.

16. **Right karate chop.** Say aloud, "This depression," followed by a **deep inhale and a sigh**.

    Bring all four of your fingertips back to the meaty portion of the right hand. Tap right on the meaty portion. Take a nice deep inhale and give yourself permission to make the biggest sigh you've done all day. Repeat that huge inhale and sigh a second time.

    Shake out your tapping hands. That was a full round of tapping. Think back on that same memory and measure the intensity of the depression from 0 to 10. Note what it was at the beginning of the round. How do the two numbers compare? It could be down to 0 already, still at a 9/10, or anywhere in between. For the purposes of this example, let's say the feeling of depression went down from a 9/10 to a 5/10.

What Do You Do If You Still Have Some Intensity?

Edit the opening statement and reminder phrase:
1. This remaining _____.
2. This little bit of _____.
3. This tiny sliver of _____.

You will edit the opening statement and the reminder phrase. We completed one full round of tapping. We still have some of the depression feeling left (5/10), so we want to continue to work with it. You would do additional tapping rounds until the feeling had been completely integrated, changing the opening statement and reminder phrase for each round and repeating the full tapping round just like we did above. We signal to our subconscious what it is that we're working on now. This is how you work with any remaining intensity. The goal is to bring the intensity down to 0 or as close as possible.

For our second round, we would use the phrase "Even though I am feeling this remaining depression, I deeply and profoundly love and accept myself. Our reminder phrase would be "this remaining depression."

Let's say you had done that, and the feeling of depression went from a 5/10 to a 1/10. You would then do a third round. Your next opening statement would be "Even though I am feeling this little bit of depression, I deeply and profoundly love and accept myself." Your new reminder phrase would be "this little bit of depression."

Let's say you had completed the third round using those phrases and there was still a .25/10 at that point, you would then do a fourth round. The opening statement would be "Even though I'm feeling this tiny sliver of <u>depression</u>, I deeply and profoundly love and accept myself." The reminder phrase would be "this tiny sliver of <u>depression</u>."

Additive Tapping

We want to use this technique after doing reductive tapping (Dawson & Marillat, 2014). By doing reductive tapping first as in the example above, what we've done is bring love and acceptance to what's already here. That caused us to have an emotional shift. In this example, we brought love and acceptance to the feeling of depression. Ideally, you would continue tapping through the depression until it was at a 0. Then you would do the additive tapping process.

When we do additive tapping, we're inviting in something related to whatever we had just tapped on. In this case, we tapped on depression. What we want to do is to invite in something that feels better to us than depression. For depression, we might choose to bring in more joy, energy, ease, lightness, etc. Some examples could be if we tapped on anger because you weren't feeling safe, or sadness because you weren't showing up as authentically as you'd like. Then we would do an additive tapping process around these things because we had tapped through an issue that concerned the absence of these things. In other words, if you're angry because you're lacking safety, you want to invite in more safety. If you're sad because you weren't showing up authentically, you want to invite in more authenticity. If you processed the anger using the reductive tapping process above, then you want to invite in more safety in this round.

Additive tapping phrases
1. I wonder what it would be like if . . .
2. I can . . .
3. I am choosing to . . .
4. I am . . .

When you do additive tapping, these are the phrases to call in what you want. These allow us to get our imagination and our subconscious on board. By tapping through the points and saying things in this order through steps 1, 2, 3, and 4, we're going from less certain to more certain, from less strong to stronger. Let's look at an example of safety. We could tap through the points above and start with "I wonder what it would be like if I felt safer in my body. I can feel safer in my body. I am choosing to feel safer in my body. I am safer in my body." Then we would go through and tap through the rest of the points. We would choose phrases that also have to do with cultivating more safety in our lives. We can also continue to use these phrases throughout the remaining tapping process.

Additive Tapping Process: Feeling Better

Since we've just worked through depression earlier, let's invite in something that might feel better than that. You'll see that additive tapping is much more adlibbed. We make it up as we go along, based on whatever it is that wants to come through and whatever flows naturally. Reductive tapping is very formulaic. It follows a set way of doing things just to make it easy. Additive tapping is created in an improvised way.

Follow the process below to experience an additive tapping example. Begin by noticing how you feel now, and then begin the round below.

The First Half of the Additive Practice Round

1. **Left karate chop.** Say aloud, "I wonder what it would be like if I felt better," followed by a **deep inhale and a sigh.**

   Take your left hand and extend it in a karate chop as if you're about to chop wood. Take the four fingertips of the right hand and bring them to the karate chop area of the left hand. Make sure you're tapping on the meaty portion of the hand with your fingertips.

2. **Eyebrow.** Say aloud, "I can feel better," followed by a **deep inhale and a sigh.**

   Bring the two index and the middle fingertips of both hands to the furry part of the eyebrows, right where they meet the nose. Tap there for a few moments.

3. **Side of the eye.** Say aloud, "I am choosing to feel better," followed by a **deep inhale and a sigh.**

   Then tap on the temples, which are outside the eyebrows. You can feel there's a small indentation in the skull. Tap there.

4. **Cheekbone.** Say aloud, "I am feeling better," followed by a **deep inhale and a sigh.**

   Tap on the cheekbones directly below the eyes. Your fingers should be directly in line with your eyes.

   As you go through these tapping processes, sighs, yawns, and other noises may naturally emerge. These are part of the release process, so allow them to move through.

5. **Upper lip.** Say aloud, "When I feel down, I take care of myself. I do the best I can to meet myself where I am," followed by a **deep inhale and a sigh.**

   With the fingertips of the index and middle fingers of one hand, tap below the nose in the crevice in the upper lip.

6. **Lower lip.** Say aloud, "When I feel down, I do things to help myself feel better," followed by a **deep inhale and a sigh.**

   Now tap in the crevice above the chin and below the bottom lip.

7. **Collarbone.** Say aloud, "I am choosing to take care of myself," followed by a **deep inhale and a sigh.**

   Now we're going to find the collarbone point. To me, this is the most difficult point to find. Feel your collarbones at the top of your chest. Below your collarbones is a hollow area. You can feel the sternum there as well, running up and down. Using your dominant hand, place your thumb on one side of it and your index and middle finger on the other side. You'll know it's the right place because it's soft there. Make sure that your thumb, index, and middle fingers are as close to your sternum as possible. Tap there for a moment.

Make sure you're not tapping so softly that you can't feel it. Make sure you're not being unkind to yourself by tapping too hard.

8. **Heart.** Say aloud, "I am choosing to do the things that are going to help me feel good," followed by a **deep inhale and a sigh**.

   Place all four fingertips of your tapping hand right on your sternum above the heart. Tap there.

9. **Armpit.** Say aloud, "When I honor myself and take care of myself, I feel better," followed by a **deep inhale and a sigh**.

   Now tap on the armpit points. This is four inches below your armpits. Tap around in this area and see if there are any tender spots. If there are tender spots, tap right on them. If not, tap four inches below your armpits.

10. **Solar plexus.** Say aloud, "When I feel depressed, it can be hard for me to take care of myself," followed by a **deep inhale and a sigh**.

    Find your solar plexus at the base of the ribs. Tap from the center of your bottom ribs out along the bottom ribs toward your sides. See if you can find any tender spots there. If you find any tender spots, tap right on them. If not, you can tap directly in line with the nipples.

11. **Left wrist.** Say aloud, "When I feel depressed, I sometimes don't feel worthy of taking care of myself," followed by a **deep inhale and a sigh.**

    Extend your left hand palm up toward the sky. Take the two fingertips of your right hand and tap on the center of the left wrist right where it meets the hand.

12. **Side of the left thumb.** Say aloud, "When I feel depressed, it can be hard for me to muster the energy to take care of myself," followed by a **deep inhale and a sigh.**

    Then tap on the side of the left thumb, right by the nail, not on the nail or the underside of the finger. If you were to try to chop a piece of wood, this would be the part of your thumb that is facing toward the ceiling. Make sure you're using your fingertips.

    Make sure you're using your fingertips to tap directly on each point.

13. **Side of the left index finger.** Say aloud, "I choose to take care of myself anyway," followed by a **deep inhale and a sigh.**

    Tap on the side of the index finger on the same spot. Tap right on the side where the nail is but not on the nail.

14. **Side of the left middle finger.** Say aloud, "I know that as long as I take care of myself, eventually I'll feel better," followed by a **deep inhale and a sigh.**

    Repeat with the middle finger.

Keep your left hand still and just move your right hand. Leave the tapping fingers of the right hand extended as you rotate the tapping hand palm up toward the ceiling.

15. **Underside of the left ring finger.** Say aloud, "Emotions come and go," followed by a **deep inhale and a sigh**.

    Bring the fingertips onto the underside of your ring finger by the nail. If you were chopping wood with your left hand, it would be the side of your ring finger facing the ground.

16. **Underside of the left pinky finger.** Say aloud, "Emotions are temporary," followed by a **deep inhale and a sigh**.

    Continue tapping on the same spot on the pinky finger.

17. **Left karate chop.** Say aloud, "I remember that this too shall pass," followed by a **deep inhale, huge sigh**. "This too shall pass." **Deep inhale, huge sigh.**

    Bring all four of your fingertips back to the meaty portion of the left hand. Tap right on the meaty portion.

Practicing the 9-Gamut Procedure

Take the two fingertips of your right hand and find the knuckles of your left ring finger and pinky finger. Place your two fingertips there. Trace your fingertips back toward the wrist about an inch higher than the knuckles. You'll find a hollow area there. Place the fingertips of your index and middle fingers there. Tap here for the remainder of the 9-Gamut Procedure (Craig & Fowlie, 1995).

1. Keep your chin parallel to the floor. Don't move your head throughout this process. Continue to tap on this point.
2. Keeping your head still, look down to the left.
3. Look down to the right.
4. Roll the eyes fully one way.
5. Roll the eyes fully the other way.
6. Count to five out loud.
7. Hum a tune for a few seconds.

    I like to use "Oh, When the Saints." Use a real tune instead of making one up.

8. Count to seven out loud.
9. Hum a tune again.

The Second Half of the Additive Practice Round

1. **Eyebrow.** Say aloud, "I am choosing to feel better," followed by a **deep inhale and a sigh.**

    Bring the two index and the middle fingertips of both hands to the furry part of the eyebrows, right where they meet the nose. Tap there for a few moments.

2. **Side of the eye.** Say aloud, "I know that even though I feel depressed sometimes, I'm not going to feel that way forever," followed by a **deep inhale and a sigh.**

Then tap on the temples, which are outside the eyebrows. You can feel there's a small indentation in the skull. Tap there.

3. **Cheekbone.** Say aloud, "Like all feelings, this feeling is here now, but it will not be here forever," followed by a **deep inhale and a sigh**.

   Tap on the cheekbones directly below the eyes. Your fingers should be directly in line with your eyes.

4. **Upper lip.** Say aloud, "I remember the good things in life," followed by a **deep inhale and a sigh**.

   With the fingertips of the index and middle fingers of one hand, tap below the nose in the crevice in the upper lip.

5. **Lower lip.** Say aloud, "Even though it's hard for me to see those good things now, I know that I've felt them before," followed by a **deep inhale and a sigh**.

   Now tap in the crevice above the chin and below the bottom lip.

6. **Collarbone.** Say aloud, "I'm doing the best that I can," followed by a **deep inhale and a sigh**.

   Now we're going to find the collarbone point. To me, this is the most difficult point to find. Feel your collarbones at the top of your chest. Below your collarbones is a hollow area. You can feel the sternum there as well, running up and down. Using your dominant hand, place your thumb on one side of it and your index and middle finger on the other side. You'll know it's the right spot because it's soft there. Make sure that your thumb, index, and middle fingers are as close to your sternum as possible. Tap there for a moment.

7. **Heart.** Say aloud, "I am taking care of myself," followed by a **deep inhale and a sigh.**

   Place all four fingertips of your tapping hand right on your sternum above the heart. Tap there.

8. **Armpit.** Say aloud, "When I take care of myself, I win," followed by a **deep inhale and a sigh.**

   Now tap on the armpit points. This is four inches below your armpits. Tap around in this area and see if you can find any tender spots. If there are tender spots, tap right on them. If not, tap four inches below your armpits.

9. **Solar plexus.** Say aloud, "When I take care of myself, I send a signal to my system," followed by a **deep inhale and a sigh.**

   Find your solar plexus at the base of the ribs. Tap from the center of your bottom ribs out along the bottom ribs toward your sides. See if you can find any tender spots there. If you find any tender spots, tap right on them. If not, you can tap directly in line with the nipples.

10. **Right wrist.** Say aloud, "I signal to my system that I am worthy," followed by a **deep inhale and a sigh.**

    Extend your right hand palm up toward the sky. Take the two fingertips of your left hand and tap on the center of the right wrist right where it meets the hand.

11. **Side of the right thumb.** Say aloud, "When I take care of myself, I tell my system that even though I'm not feeling good right now, I'm still worthy," followed by a **deep inhale and a sigh.**

    Then tap on the side of the right thumb by the nail, not on the nail or the underside of the finger. If you were to try to chop a piece of wood, this would be the part of your thumb that is facing toward the ceiling.

    Make sure you're using your fingertips to tap directly on each point.

12. **Side of the right index finger.** Say aloud, "I am worthy of caring for myself. I am worthy of being taken care of," followed by a **deep inhale and a sigh.**

    Tap on the side of the index finger on the same spot. Tap on the side where the nail is but not on the nail.

13. **Side of the right middle finger:** Say aloud, "I am worthy at all times. There is no time and no moment in which I am unworthy," followed by a **deep inhale and a sigh.**

    Repeat with the middle finger.

    Keep your right hand still and just move your left hand. Leave the tapping fingers of the left hand extended as you rotate the tapping hand palm up toward the ceiling.

14. **Underside of the right ring finger.** Say aloud, "When I take care of myself, I provide the fertile ground for my system to restore itself. When I take care of myself, I am lovingly inviting myself back home to a state of well-being.

I absolutely love taking care of myself. When I do that, I am better able to experience the love and beauty of the world," followed by a **deep inhale and a sigh.**

Bring the fingertips onto the underside of your ring finger by the nail. If you were chopping wood with your right hand, it would be the side of your ring finger facing the ground.

15. **Underside of the right pinky finger.** Say aloud, "Even taking time to do this tapping process is me taking care of myself," followed by a **deep inhale and a sigh.**

Continue tapping on the same spot on the pinky finger.

16. **Right karate chop.** Say aloud, "And so I remember that this too shall pass." **Deep inhale, huge sigh.** "And I take care of myself to restore and maintain my well-being. I do what I need to, to restore and maintain my well-being," followed by a **deep inhale and huge sigh.**

Bring all four of your fingertips to the meaty portion of the right hand. Tap right on the meaty portion. Take a nice deep inhale and give yourself permission to make the biggest sigh you've done all day. Repeat that huge inhale and sigh a second time.

Shake out your tapping hands. Take note of how you are feeling after practicing this additive tapping process.

When to Use Tapping

When you notice yourself having a difficult emotion (Singh, 2015), you can go through a reductive tapping process. If you need help putting a name on the emotion that you're working with, you can access the feelings inventory below, and you'll get the awesome feelings inventory I referred to earlier. Be sure to measure the intensity of the emotion if you're doing a reductive tapping process from 0 to 10 before you start. Go through the process and measure again at the end. As you practice, you'll be able to finish a round of reductive tapping in five to 15 minutes.

Go to www.bit.ly/PTSDHealing to access the feelings inventory. Use Messenger keyword: feelings inventory.

You can use additive tapping after doing reductive tapping or on its own to bolster yourself and bring in more positivity. However, if you're having a difficult experience, I recommend working through that first before doing any additive tapping. As far as inviting in what you would like, if you need some ideas, use the needs inventory below. This will give you some inspiration as far as what you might want to invite more of. When you're doing an additive tapping process, allow yourself to get creative. Tune into yourself and notice what it is you really want. Allow yourself to express and give voice to that. Additive tapping varies in length. You can do a quick round of that or really flesh it out and get nuanced and detailed like we've done above.

Go to www.bit.ly/PTSDHealing to access the needs inventory. Use Messenger keyword: needs inventory.

Considerations

Tapping is not something that we see people do very frequently in public. You will likely want to find some space to tap in a comfortable environment.

You can tap on your hand points as a way of calming yourself more discreetly while you're with people. If you're in a meeting, you can discreetly tap by keeping your hands in your lap. You can tap through the hand points while incorporating the breath, and no one will know that you're doing that. Be sure to avoid sighing if you choose to do this in that setting. Instead, take some deep breaths quietly as you go through each point. This is a way you can take care of yourself while you're with other people.

Tapping Has No Contraindications

There are no conditions or situations where tapping is not recommended. You can use it as often as you'd like, and there haven't been any issues associated with the practice as far as research is concerned.

Surface versus Underlying Causes and Triggers

Let's discuss surface versus underlying causes and triggers. I conceptualize issues in two different ways. We have certain things which are temporary, passing, and not recurring. Then we have certain deeper elements like triggers that are recurring or have a pattern. For recurring things like triggers or health issues, we want to go to the root of those issues (Dawson & Allenby, 2010). Recall that in the first full practice round of tapping, I invited you to think about to the most difficult memory from the past week. We then tapped on that memory and cleared the charge of the dominant emotion. Healing deeper issues is extremely similar in terms of resolving the root of something.

For example, someone close to me had vertigo. I had her recall the top three memories in which her vertigo was the most intense. We started to work through her most intense memory related to the vertigo. I had her start to tell the story of that experience. I asked her what the most prominent symptom was. In her case, it was dizziness. We then used the same reductive tapping processes we went through in this chapter. We brought it down to zero over several rounds, and then she could recall this memory without having any dizziness symptoms occurring. We did that for the three most intense memories related to the vertigo. It took about 90 minutes to go through the stories for all three memories. Afterward, the vertigo did not return for months because we had shown her subconscious that something else was possible by showing it that the symptoms didn't have to be permanent.

Think back to when the condition was at its worst. You can tap on the symptoms using the same phrases that we've gone over today to clear and integrate them. As a result, we often feel better and can have lasting results. I cannot, however, make blanket statements or promise miracles, so consider this my disclaimer.

Let's go deeper for a moment. In the example above, the vertigo came back after some months. This was because, while we cleared the dizziness charge from the memories, other underlying causes were not addressed. In other words, she did not investigate or alleviate any other mental or emotional factors that were contributing to the vertigo. As a result, the vertigo returned after several months.

Go to www.bit.ly/PTSDHealing to access the cheat sheet and chapter 2 summary. Use Messenger keyword: chapter two cheat sheet.

Chapter Two Brief Summary

- There are two types of Tapping; additive and reductive.
- Reductive Tapping is how we release the emotional charge.
- Additive Tapping is how we bring in positive beliefs with Tapping. This is best done after reductive Tapping.
- The Tapping points combined with bilateral stimulation bring the brain, body, and energy systems fully online to move the stuck energy through.
- The opening statement and reminder phrase signal our subconscious mind about what it is we are working with.

For full video support and expert guidance to clear out the traumatic charge and bring in new positive beliefs, join us for the Clear My PTSD Healing Accelerator at www.ClearMyPTSD.com/course

CHAPTER 3:

STOP THE NIGHTMARES, INTRUSIVE THOUGHTS, AND TRIGGERS FOR GOOD— HOW TO USE TAPPING TO DRASTICALLY REDUCE PTSD AT ITS CORE SO YOU CAN MOVE ON WITH YOUR LIFE

In This Chapter

In this chapter, we're going to cover the importance of creating safety and how to actively create it. Then we'll make a list of traumatic memories and explore how to clear the emotional intensity from them. After that, we'll look at clearing any residual feelings from those traumatic memories followed by the implications for PTSD symptoms. Lastly, we'll focus on bringing in the positive.

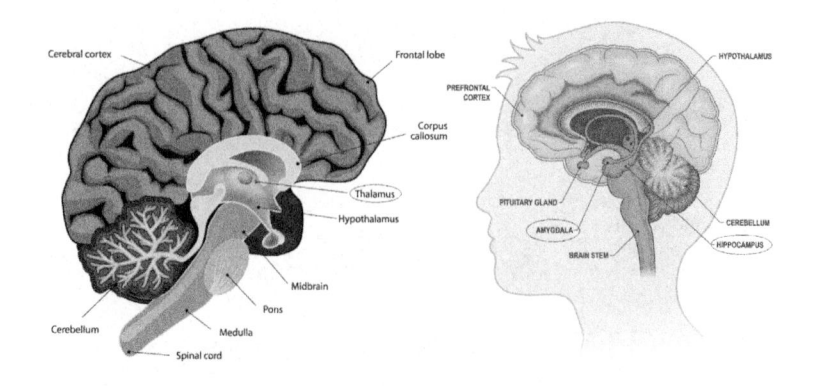

Trauma and Safety

Figure 13. Trauma and safety in the brain.

A Biological and Emotional Perspective

As we spoke about in chapter one, the brain takes in sensory information—sight, sound, taste, and touch—through the thalamus (van der Kolk, 2014). As that information comes in, it gets filtered through the amygdala, which labels it with emotion keywords (figure 13). If the information seems sad, the amygdala puts a sad stamp on it, categorizing it as sad. If anger seems like the dominant emotion in the event, the amygdala will categorize it as angry. Generally, memories then move on to the hippocampus, the hard drive of the brain where they're stored in memory. However, with trauma, the memories don't necessarily move into the hippocampus. They hang out by the amygdala. This is what allows them to get retriggered when additional sensory information is processed by the thalamus. That's when what you may be seeing, hearing, or touching remind you of the trauma. The trauma hasn't been put in storage. It's hanging out by the amygdala where it's easily accessible, and that's what allows us to be retriggered. We don't feel safe because of our ability to get so easily retriggered. It's very hard for us to relax because we're on edge as a result of these unprocessed memories. Tapping helps us clear the charge, allowing the memory to move into storage so the nervous system can relax and we feel safer.

An Energetic Perspective

From an Eastern medicine perspective and the tapping perspective, all disease—physical, mental, emotional, or spiritual—is caused by a block in the flow of energy through the body. Energy flows through via meridian lines, which are like electrical lines that bring the energy to all the different parts of the body (Solomon, 2007). That's what allows us to sustain our health and well-being. When that energy gets disrupted, that's what causes illness. That's what trauma is—the stuck energy. This is what causes us to feel unsafe. With tapping, we are getting this energy unstuck and restoring its flow.

We can see from both the biological brain and energetic perspectives that stuck energy is what's keeping us feeling unsafe and causing us to have difficulty relaxing.

Trauma in the Chakras

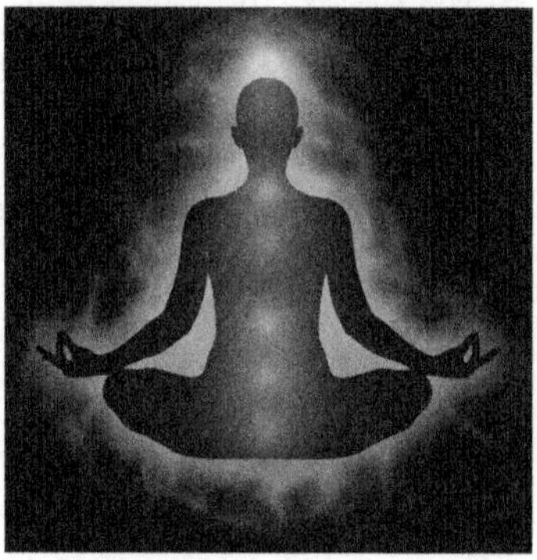

Figure 14. The chakra system.

Trauma affects the root chakra. We all have seven chakras, which are energy centers in the body that govern different life issues. The root chakra governs safety and security (Judith & Jenner, 2016). When trauma occurs, our sense of safety and security is disrupted. The root chakra is also the closest to the earth. When our root chakra is open and activated, it allows us to ground and feel connected to the earth. When we're ungrounded, we start to feel anxiety because we're no longer tethered and anchored to the earth properly. The root chakra and our ability to be grounded is part of what helps us to be present in our lives. When trauma happens, often we feel unsafe being present in the here and now. There's a subconscious fear that what happened may happen again. Perhaps we don't like being here because we have to feel the discomfort of the trauma stored in the body, so we want to leave. We leave the present moment and become depressed—stuck in the past or worried about the future.

Trauma and Addiction

We use addiction to cover over the pain and discomfort of being present. Whether the addiction is drugs, alcohol, sex, or television, it helps us avoid having to deal with the pain and discomfort of being here now.

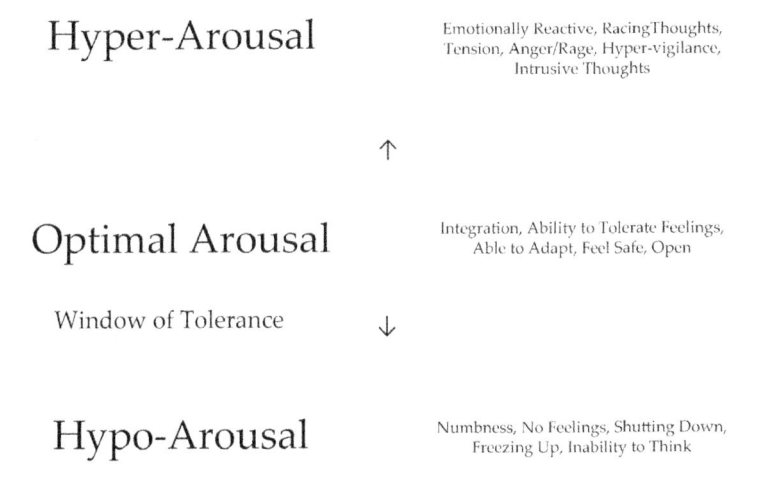

Hyper-Arousal — Emotionally Reactive, Racing Thoughts, Tension, Anger/Rage, Hyper-vigilance, Intrusive Thoughts

↑

Optimal Arousal — Integration, Ability to Tolerate Feelings, Able to Adapt, Feel Safe, Open

Window of Tolerance   ↓

Hypo-Arousal — Numbness, No Feelings, Shutting Down, Freezing Up, Inability to Think

The Most Important Reason to Create Safety: The Window of Tolerance

Figure 15. The window of tolerance.

The window of tolerance is the most important reason for safety when we're doing trauma work (Siegel, 2012). In the middle, there is what's called optimal arousal (figure 15). The middle box is also called the window of tolerance; this is what we're able to tolerate. We've talked earlier about sensory information coming into the brain. If we're able to tolerate what it is that we're experiencing, we stay in the window of tolerance.

If we start getting agitated and anxious, we get what's called *hyperarousal*. This is where we become emotionally reactive and snap at people. This is also where we start to feel anger, rage, and become hypervigilant, constantly on guard for danger.

We can also go in the other direction—toward the bottom—which is *hypoarousal*. You can think of this as underarousal where we numb out, freeze, or shut down to cope with the situation.

We want to be able to maintain a sense of safety while we're doing trauma work by staying in this window of tolerance. Otherwise, if we venture into hypoarousal or hyperarousal, we have to stop doing any healing. If that happens, we're unable to be lucid and present enough to do meaningful work and experience the healing benefits. Safety is super important to help us stay in that window of tolerance.

How to Create Safety: Resourcing

Resourcing is exactly what it sounds like. It's where we give the system what it needs to have its needs met and to relax (Spiers, 2001). With trauma, the system is often underresourced. Meaning, the way that we experience this is feeling like we don't have the tools to cope. We feel unsafe, but we don't know what to do to create safety. It's like if I ask you to make a peanut butter and jelly sandwich, but you don't know where the bread or the peanut butter or the jelly is, and you don't know what a knife is.

Many Different Ways to Resource Yourself

1.	Having a cup of tea
2.	Taking a bath
3.	Getting enough sleep
4.	Taking breaks
5.	Eating healthy and staying hydrated
6.	Making sure food, water, and bathroom access are available
7.	Creating connection with another person
8.	Practicing meditation and guided meditation

These are some different ways to resource yourself (Spiers, 2001). Notice that there are two main themes here. Having a cup of tea and taking a bath and meditation all help to relax the system. Getting enough sleep, eating healthy, and making sure that food, water, shelter, and bathroom access are available all have to do with making sure that our basic needs are met. These basic needs correspond to the root chakra that we've looked at earlier. When those basic needs are met, our system innately feels safer. As a result, we can do more in our lives, and we can do healing work as well.

Guided Meditation

The main method that I like for resourcing is guided meditation. It's something you can do when you have your phone with you or if you have access to a laptop. It's something you could do while you're sitting and you have a few minutes at home, on a bus, or in a public setting. All you need are headphones. Guided meditation is where someone uses his or her voice to guide you through a process with a specific intention, usually by visualizing certain things (Call, 2010). Guided meditation can be used to relax, to meet your spirit guide or higher self, or to create safety. I like guided meditation for resourcing because it's very intentional. We are going into it with the intention of creating safety, and it gives us a designated activity to do that on a daily basis and during trauma work. It's something we can incorporate directly into the healing work, compared to something like drawing a bath where we have to run the water and wait a little while. For tea, we have to have the tea, a cup, and access to hot water. As long as we have a phone or a laptop, we can do a guided meditation at any time while we're working through trauma.

A Guided Meditation for Safety

1.	What is a safe place for you?	
	a.	Examples: the beach, the forest, your grandma's house when you were a kid
	b.	Mine is a creek with hot spring pools next to it.
	c.	Describe the place in as much detail as you can.
2.	Who is in this safe place?	
	a.	It could be anyone: relatives alive or passed, spirit guides, religious figures, etc.
	b.	In mine are Jesus, Mother Mary, Saint Germain, my spirit guides.
	c.	Describe the people there in as much detail as you can.

To create a guided meditation for you to embody safety, grab a piece of paper and a pen, and **write down what a safe place is for you** (Spiers, 2001). Some examples might be the beach, the forest, or your grandmother's house when you were a kid. Mine is a creek with hot spring pools next to it. Also **write down who you would like to have present with you in your safe place** (Spiers, 2001).

Here is an example from a client (figure 16):

A. Place:	B. People:
1. The ocean	1. Tribal people of the land
2. Sounds of the waves	2. Grandma—a guide
3. Warmth of the sun	3. Their dog
4. Beach blanket	
5. Pillows	
6. Riding in the waves/swimming	
7. Dense forests behind back	
8. Mountains in the distance	
9. Soft ground in the forest to be able to walk barefoot comfortably	

Figure 16. Examples of places and people for resourcing meditation.

Resourcing Meditation Practice Process

Go to www.bit.ly/PTSDHealing to access the resourcing meditation video, template, and script. Use Messenger keyword: resourcing meditation

    I want to invite you now to close your eyes if that feels safe and comfortable. If not, you can leave them cracked, looking with a gentle gaze down at the floor a few feet in front of you. Begin to pay attention to the sensation of your breath coming in and out through your nose. Feel the sensation coming in, going out, in and out.

    In your mind's eye, see yourself standing in a *grassy field*. You can feel the texture of the *grass* between your toes. You can hear the sounds of the *birds chirping in the trees* and smell the *wildflowers* on the breeze.

    The sun shines down gently, comfortably from above. As the sunlight touches your face and head, all negative energy begins to melt away from there, collecting in a puddle on the ground by your feet. The sunlight flows down your body, melting away all the negative energy from your neck, torso, arms, and hands. This too collects in a puddle on the ground. Finally, the sunlight touches your waist, legs, and feet, melting away all the negative energy from there. This energy drips down into the puddle on the ground.

    You walk forward, leaving this puddle behind as you explore this beautiful, safe place. You approach a creek off to your right, sitting down by the water's edge. *Hearing the sound of the water*, you find yourself relaxing more and more.

As you sit, *Mother Mary* emerges from the field behind you, placing her hands on your shoulders, cradling you. You can feel the love, compassion, and safety emanating from her.

This safety begins to enter every cell in your body. See every cell of your body glow with the energy of safety. You *are* safe. You *are* safe. You feel this energy glowing so strongly that you know if you opened your eyes and looked in a mirror, you would see yourself glowing with it. You could see it glowing through your skin.

This energy goes even deeper within your being, settling into your very bones. Your bones now glow with the energy of safety. The feeling of safety settles into your very bones. You know that you are safe. You say to yourself, "I *am* safe. I *am* safe."

You feel yourself settle into your body, allowing yourself to be more present, more whole, more here.

Breathe into this sense of safety. Breathe into this sense of presence and wholeness.

As you settle into this feeling, you notice that there is a violet flame around you. This violet flame feels entirely safe and entirely comfortable. This violet flame enters every cell of your body. Every cell of your body is glowing with the violet flame so strongly that if you opened your eyes and looked in a mirror, you would see it glowing through your skin.

This violet flame breaks down all negative energy in your entire body at the particle level. These particles are extracted through your skin. See these particles now, glowing with the violet flame energy. See them transformed into positive, supportive energy, perhaps changing to a golden color. See this positive, supportive energy fall away, down past your feet, into the soil, nourishing the earth with this positive, supportive energy.

This violet flame expands to encompass your entire body and your aura, going three feet out on all sides. This violet flame breaks down all negative energy in your entire body and your aura at the particle level. These particles are extracted through your skin. See these particles now, glowing with the violet flame energy. See them transformed into positive, supportive energy, perhaps changing to a golden color. See this positive, supportive energy fall away, down past your feet, into the soil, nourishing the earth with this positive, supportive energy.

This violet flame expands again to encompass your entire body, your aura, and your field, going 25 feet out on all sides. This violet flame breaks down all negative energy in your body, your aura, and your field at the particle level. These particles are extracted through your skin. See these particles now, glowing with the violet flame energy. See them transformed into positive, supportive energy, perhaps changing to a golden color. See this positive, supportive energy fall away, down past your feet, into the soil, nourishing the earth with this positive, supportive energy.

Notice how you feel now. Notice the embodied sense of safety. Breathe into this newfound way of being. Thank *Mother Mary*. Thank whoever else came to assist you. Thank the land for supporting this process.

Start to notice the sensations in your body. Notice your breath. Taking your time, at your own pace, come back and open your eyes.

Meditation Script Example

This is a resourcing meditation script that I created. The things that I've italicized have to do with the environment or the people in the meditation. You can replace these italicized things with the things you came up with for your safe space. You can replace this grassy field with whatever your environment was, whether it was the beach, the forest, or something else. The birds chirping in the trees could be replaced with the sound of the ocean. You might replace the grass with the feeling of sand and the wildflowers with the smell of the ocean. Mother Mary could be replaced with Grandma, Jesus, Buddha, Krishna, or whoever feels right to you. Whatever it is that's going to give you a sense of safety is what you want to substitute in place of what I've listed here. All you do is plug and play. Plug in your people and details into these italicized spots replacing what's there. Then you'll have your own resourcing meditation.

Meditation Script Next Steps

1.	Plug in your own place details and people.
2.	Once the script is complete, record yourself reading it.
3.	Then
	a. Try it for once to see how you feel. Tweak as needed.
	b. Try it once per day for a week.
	c. Try it for 30 days and see if there's a lasting difference.

Once your script is complete and you've plugged your information in, take out your phone and open up the voice memo app. Record yourself reading your script. You'll then have a guided meditation in your own voice. When you've done that, you can try it once to see how you feel afterward. Then you can tweak the script as needed and rerecord if that's something that feels helpful. The main goal of trying it once is just to see how you feel after doing it. If it feels beneficial, you can try it once per day for a week and see how you feel after doing it repeatedly. Then if it feels beneficial having done it for a week, try it for 30 days and see if there's a lasting impact. By doing this regularly, you are retraining your body and your system to know what safety feels like. You're creating a new baseline in your system from which to operate. You'll see shortly how this fits into the rest of the trauma healing work.

Making a List of Your Traumatic Memories

1.	Do the resourcing guided meditation.
2.	Take out a piece of paper and a pen.
3.	List out up to 20 traumatic memories:
	a. Memories that influence your experience of PTSD
	b. Give them brief names—up to five words or a sentence.
4.	If you need to take a break during this, honor and take care of yourself.

Go to www.bit.ly/PTSDHealing to access the traumatic memory list template. Use Messenger keyword: traumatic memory list.

Now that you have a sense of how to create safety, let's look at how to work through trauma with tapping. After doing the resourcing meditation, take out your pen and paper and list out up to 20 traumatic memories. Give them brief names using up to five words or a sentence (Church, 2017). Notice that the first instruction is to do the resourcing guided meditation. This puts your system in the space of relaxation before doing this exercise. Writing down your traumatic memories can bring up some intensity and anxiety. If you resource yourself before doing that, you are buffering yourself against the intensity that might come up while you list the stuff out. The 20 memories you are writing down are the ones most influencing your experience of PTSD. You don't have to have 20, but you can write down up to 20. If you have more than 20, you can list out however many you have. If you're having dreams, nightmares, or intrusive thoughts about certain experiences, this would be where you list out the memories that are responsible for those things. If you need to take a little break while you're listing them out, please take care of yourself. It's really important that you honor yourself and take care of yourself.

Memory List Example and Process

Rank	Memory name	Starting intensity (0-10)	Ending intensity (0-10)
2	Goldilocks and the Three Bears	9	0
5	Aladdin	6	0
1	The Three Little Pigs	10	0

| 3 | Cinderella | 8 | 0 |
| 4 | Little Red Riding Hood | 7 | 0 |

Figure 17. Memory list examples.

I've put in the names of some fairy tales in place of memory names (figure 17). Feel into the emotional intensity of each memory from 0 to 10 and put a number down to the right of each memory for the emotional intensity. Intensity ranges from 0 to 10. Put the emotional intensity score for each of the memories on your list.

Once you've got those emotional intensity scores written down, to the left of each memory name, number them from 1 (having the greatest intensity) up to 20 (having the least intensity). Any memories that you have that are at a 10/10 will be labeled first. Any memories that you have that are at a 9/10 would be labeled 2 and so on. Memories labeled 1 will be the most intense; 2 would be the second most intense; 3 would be the third most intense; and so on. Organize them by numbering them from greatest to least intensity: 1 being most intense and 20 being least intense. Later, as you clear the charge from each memory, return to the list and write in the ending intensity.

Clearing the Charge of the Intensity and Remaining Emotions:

The Window of Tolerance Revisited

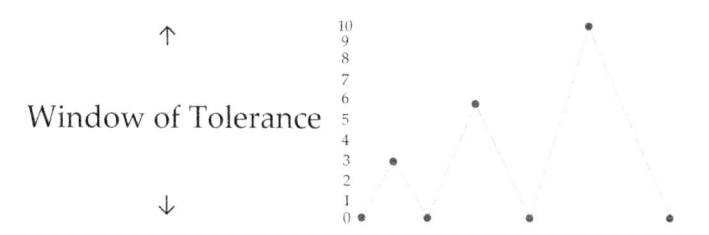

Window of Tolerance

Earlier, we've looked at the window of tolerance. When we're healing trauma, it's super important that we stay in that window (Siegel, 2012). We don't want to go above it and activate our fight-or-flight response, and we don't want to go below it and activate our freeze response.

Now we'll bring in the window of tolerance and look at how to work with these memories. Let's start with your most intense memory.

The Window of Tolerance: 3/10

Window of Tolerance

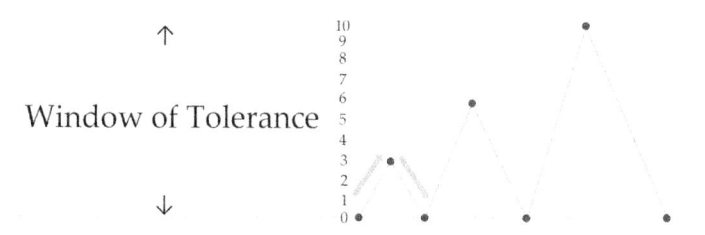

First, what we'll do is start at 0. At that point, we would do the resourcing meditation, and then we would start to tell the story of that memory until we reached a 3/10 in intensity. Even if the memory is at a 10/10 or something in total intensity or at 9/10 or 11/10, we would still only tell the story until we've reached a

3/10. Then we would use tapping to bring that 3/10 back down to a 0.

We would use the resourcing meditation again to make sure we're coming back down to our baseline again at 0. (Levine, 2012).

Then we would start to tell the story again from the beginning until we reached a 6/10 in intensity. Once we got to a 6/10, we would use tapping to bring the intensity down to a 0 again. Practice the resourcing meditation again here.

Then we would tell the story again from the beginning until we got to a 10/10 in intensity. Then we would use tapping to bring that 10/10 down to a 0. Do the resourcing meditation again afterward.

We're never leaving the window of tolerance. Doing it this way teaches our system to be able to tolerate going in and out of these intense emotional states safely. Eventually, we can get through the whole story without having any intensity come up. We tell the story from the beginning each time: once until reaching a 3/10, once until reaching a 6/10, once until reaching a 10/10. After we do that, we would tell the story from the beginning again, restarting the process. We would repeat the cycle of 3/10, 6/10, and 10/10 each time, getting through more and more of the story with less and less intensity coming up until we can get through the whole story with no intensity showing up.

Tell the Story: Up to 3/10 Intensity

> There was once a little girl whose hair was like spun gold. Her name was Goldilocks. One day Goldilocks went out into the meadows to gather flowers. She wondered into a forest where she found a house and knocked on the door. She didn't know the house belonged to three bears: a father bear, mother bear, and baby bear. When she knocked, no one answered, so she went inside.
>
> Inside she found a table with three steaming bowls of porridge on it and three chairs around it. She tried each of the chairs. The first chair was too big, and the second chair wasn't quite right either. But the smallest chair was just right.
>
> She tried the porridge from the first bowl, but it was too hot. She tried the porridge from the second bowl, and it was too cold (Pyle, 2018).

For example, this is the story of *Goldilocks and the Three Bears*. First, you would start with the resourcing meditation. Next, tell the story until you reach a 3/10 in intensity. In this example, I only get through this paragraph before I reach that 3/10 intensity. At that point, I would stop. In other words, the story of the traumatic memory is longer than that, but I can only get up to here before I reach a 3/10, at which point I need to stop.

Use Tapping

Once I stop, then I use tapping. I notice all the feelings that I'm experiencing with this 3/10 intensity. The feelings might include anger, sadness, guilt, shame, fear, or other emotions.

Whatever those feelings are, think of those feelings together as "this intensity." Use the following opening statements as we looked at earlier. The opening statement would be "Even though I am feeling this intensity, I deeply and profoundly love and accept myself." As you're tapping through the additional tapping points, you would use the reminder phrase "this intensity" for each point. This cues your subconscious about what it is you're working on. The goal is to bring the intensity down from a 3/10 to a 0.

What Do You Do If You Still Have Some Intensity?

Opening statement	Reminder phrase
Even though I am feeling *this remaining* _____, I deeply and profoundly love and accept myself.	1. This remaining _____.
Even though I am feeling *this little bit of* _____, I deeply and profoundly love and accept myself.	2. This little bit of _____.
Even though I am feeling *this tiny sliver of* _____, I deeply and profoundly love and accept myself.	3. This tiny sliver of _____.

So let's say you did this exercise, and you still felt some intensity (anything greater than 0). You would use these phrases and adjust the opening statement and reminder phrase as needed (Church, 2017).

Examples

For example, the opening statement will become "Even though I am feeling this remaining intensity, I deeply and profoundly love and accept myself." For each point, the reminder phrase would become "this remaining intensity."

Let's say you do that, and you check in again, and you still have more intensity remaining then you would use the next phrase: "this little bit of . . ." Your opening statement would be "Even though I'm feeling this a little bit of intensity, I deeply and profoundly love and accept myself." The reminder phrase would be "this little bit of intensity." Once the intensity reaches a 0, do the resourcing meditation again or when you're done tapping through any residual feelings.

What If There Are Other Remaining Feelings?

Pain	Fear
Confusion	Anger
Guilt	Resentment
Shame	Depression
Low-Self Worth	Sadness
Anxiety	Panic

These are some really common remaining emotions for PTSD and trauma (Ellis, 2014). Let's say you notice that you still have some remaining emotions like guilt, anger, panic, etc. After you tap through the intensity, then you would tap through these emotions individually.

Tapping through the Remaining Feelings

For example, you would measure the guilt from 0 to 10. Then you would use the same format to tap through the guilt. Use the opening statement: "Even though I am feeling this guilt, I deeply and profoundly love and accept myself." Then you would tap through the points with the reminder phrase "this

113

guilt." After that, you would tap through and adjust the phrasing as needed until the guilt is a 0. In other words, you could bring in the phrasing "this remaining guilt and then this little bit of guilt" and so on until the guilt was at 0. You would do this for the other feelings as well. Once you're at 0 for all the feelings and the intensity, then practice the resourcing meditation again. Do the resourcing meditation once before telling the story and once after you've integrated and released all the emotions related to the story at the point that you stopped. In this case, the point we stopped at was 3/10.

Increasing the Intensity: 6/10

Come back to the window of tolerance. Let's take a look at what we've done so far with that initial memory. We've done the resourcing meditation. Then we told as much of the story as we could until we reached a 3/10 in intensity. We tapped out that 3/10 in intensity and any remaining feelings to bring them back to a 0. We did the resourcing meditation again to establish a baseline of safety, calm, and relaxation. Now, tell the story from the beginning until you reach a 6/10. Tap through the 6/10 and bring it back down to a 0. Do the resourcing meditation again.

Telling the Story: Up to 6/10 Intensity

> There was once a little girl whose hair was like spun gold. Her name was Goldilocks. One day Goldilocks went out into the meadows to gather flowers. She wondered into a forest where she found a house and knocked on the door. She didn't know the house belonged to three bears: a father

> bear, mother bear, and baby bear. When she knocked, no one answered, so she went inside.
>
> Inside she found a table with three steaming bowls of porridge on it and three chairs around it. She tried each of the chairs. The first chair was too big, and the second chair wasn't quite right either, but the smallest chair was just right.
>
> She tried the porridge from the first bowl, but it was too hot. She tried the porridge from the second bowl, and it was too cold (Pyle, 2018).

You're able to get further into the story. When the porridge is getting too hot is when I've reached my 6/10 in intensity. Now I've been able to get further into the story before I reach that 6/10 in intensity at which point I would stop.

You've reached a 6/10 in the story when the porridge was too hot in this example. Then, repeat the same process that you just did to tap out the 3/10 intensity. Tap out the 6/10 intensity using the same phrases. Then, tap out any residual feelings like you did for the 3/10 intensity. Then bring that 6/10 intensity down to a 0 along with any residual feelings, followed by doing the resourcing meditation again.

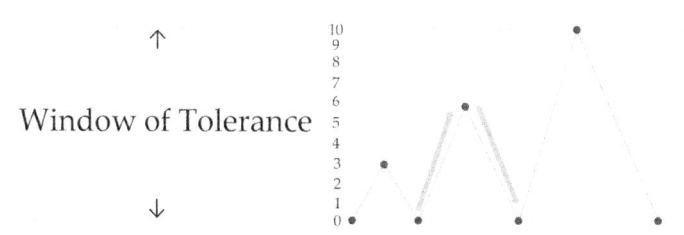

The Window of Tolerance: 6/10

At this point, you've done the resourcing meditation, told the story until you reached a 3/10, then tapped out the 3/10. Then you've done the resourcing meditation again, told the story until you reached a 6/10, gotten further into the story and then tapped out that 6/10, followed by the resourcing meditation again. Then, repeat this process again with the 10/10, meaning that you're going to tell more of the story from the beginning. You're going to be able to get further into it before you reach that 10/10 in intensity. Once you reach that 10/10, tap it out and then do the resourcing meditation again. Let's see what that looks like.

Continuing to Tell the Story: Up to a 10/10 Intensity

> There was once a little girl whose hair was like spun gold. Her name was Goldilocks. One day Goldilocks went out into the meadows to gather flowers. She wondered into a forest where she found a house and knocked on the door. She didn't know the house belonged to three bears: a father bear, mother bear, and baby bear. When she knocked, no one answered, so she went inside.
>
> Inside she found a table with three steaming bowls of porridge on it and three chairs around it. She tried each of the chairs. The first chair was too big, and the second chair wasn't quite right either, but the smallest chair was just right.
>
> She tried the porridge from the first bowl, but it was too hot. She tried the porridge from the second bowl, and it was too cold (Pyle, 2018).

Now, we've gotten past the point where the porridge is too hot. I'm able to get to this point in the story where the porridge is too cold, and that's where I reach my 10/10 in intensity, so I stop.

Tapping through This Intensity

Now, repeat the same process again that you just did for the 6/10 intensity. Use the same statements that you used to bring the 6/10 intensity down to a zero again for the 10/10. Then, tap out any residual feelings. Afterward, do the resourcing meditation again.

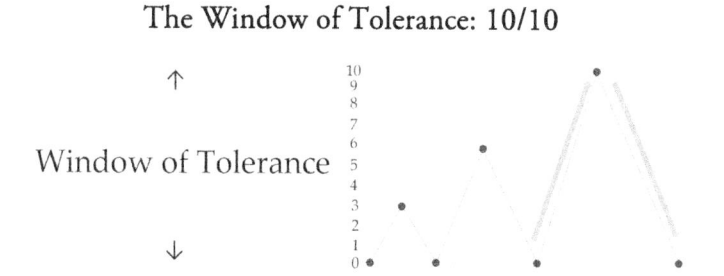

The Window of Tolerance: 10/10

Window of Tolerance

Now, you told the story until you reached a 3/10 and then tapped that out. Then you told the story until you reached a 6/10 and tapped that out. Lastly, you told the story until you reached a 10/10 and tapped that out. You did a resourcing meditation before and after each of these tapping processes. We've looked at all the opening statements and reminder phrases that we're using to help bring ourselves back down to a 0. We also looked at how to tap through any remaining feelings that we feel once we've tapped through the intensity.

Telling the Rest of the Story

> There was once a little girl whose hair was like spun gold. Her name was Goldilocks. One day Goldilocks went out into the meadows to gather flowers. She wondered into a forest where she found a house and knocked on the door. She didn't know the house belonged to three bears: a father bear, mother bear, and baby bear. When she knocked, no one answered, so she went inside.
>
> Inside she found a table with three steaming bowls of porridge on it and three chairs around it. She tried each of the chairs. The first chair was too big, and the second chair wasn't quite right either, but the smallest chair was just right.
>
> She tried the porridge from the first bowl, but it was too hot. She tried the porridge from the second bowl, and it was too cold. Lastly, she tried the smallest bowl. That porridge was just right.
>
> When she finished eating, she felt tired, and she wanted to take a nap. She wandered upstairs and found three beds. She lay down in the first bed, but that one was too soft. She lay down in the second bed, and that one was too hard. The third and smallest bed was just right. Within a few moments, she fell asleep, and the bears returned home (Pyle, 2018).

Now, tell the story from the beginning the fourth time. First, you did 3/10, then 6/10, then 10/10. Now you can get even further into it before you feel any intensity. Tell the story again from the beginning until you reach a 3/10 again. In this example, I can get up to this portion of the story where Goldilocks sat in the first chair to rest her feet before I even reach a 3/10 intensity now. So I'm getting much further into the story while having much less intensity come up. Then I would tap out this 3/10 and do the resourcing meditation again. Then I tell the story from the beginning again, and now I can get all the way to where Goldilocks fell asleep in the bed before I get to a 6/10. Now, I tap out that 6/10 and do the resourcing meditation again.

> There was once a little girl whose hair was like spun gold. Her name was Goldilocks. One day Goldilocks went out into the meadows to gather flowers. She wondered into a forest where she found a house and knocked on the door. She didn't know the house belonged to three bears: a father bear, mother bear, and baby bear. When she knocked, no one answered, so she went inside.
>
> Inside she found a table with three steaming bowls of porridge on it and three chairs around it. She tried each of the chairs. The first chair was too big, and the second chair wasn't quite right either, but the smallest chair was just right.
>
> She tried the porridge from the first bowl, but it was too hot. She tried the porridge from the second bowl, and it was too cold. Lastly, she tried the smallest bowl. That porridge was just right.
>
> When she finished eating, she felt tired, and she wanted to take a nap. She wandered upstairs and found three beds. She lay down in the first bed, but that one was too soft. She lay down in the second bed, and that one was too hard. The third and smallest bed was just right. Within a few moments, she fell asleep, and the bears returned home.
>
> "Somebody has been eating my porridge," growled the father bear. "Somebody has been eating my porridge," said the mother bear. "All my porridge is gone!" exclaimed the baby bear.
>
> "Somebody has been sitting in my chair," growled the father bear. "Somebody has been sitting in my chair," said the mother bear. "Somebody knocked my chair over!" said the baby bear.

> The three bears decided to see what was going on upstairs. When they got there, father bear roared, "Somebody's been sleeping in my bed, and now the sheets are dirty!" "Somebody's been sleeping in my bed, and they messed up the hospital corners on my sheets!" said the mother bear. "Somebody is still sleeping in my bed!" said the baby bear.
>
> Goldilocks heard them shouting and grumbling and jumped out of bed! She realized it was time to leave, so she ran from the house into the woods and never returned (Pyle, 2018).

Tell the story again from the beginning. Now I can get all the way to the very end of the story before I reach a 10/10 in intensity. Now I tap out that 10/10 in intensity, bring it down to a 0, and do the resourcing meditation again. Now I can tell the whole story without any intensity coming up after I've tapped that out, in this example. Repeat the process (3/10, 6/10, and 10/10) until you can get through the whole story with 0 intensity coming up. After tapping out that 10/10 in this example at the end of the story, then go back and tell the story from the beginning again. If any intensity comes up, tap that out as well. Always complete the resourcing meditation before telling the story and then again after tapping out any intensity.

Go through This for All Memories on the List from Most to Least Intense

At this point, you've tapped out one memory. In other words, you have cleared the emotional intensity and any residual emotions that were left over. Repeat this same process for every memory on your memory list from most intense to least intense. Start with the most intense because that's where you get the most bang for your buck.

Let's say I haven't cleaned my apartment for a while. I have a few pieces of clothing on the floor, but I cook all the time in my kitchen. As a result, I have empty jars, cans, dirty plates, pots, and utensils all over the kitchen counter. If I clean the things on the kitchen counter, the overall impact on the cleanliness of my apartment is going to be much greater than if I started by picking up the few clothing items on the floor. It's the same here. If you can clear the charge from the most intense memory first, then the second most intense memory, and then the third most intense memory, you're going to impact your system very quickly.

Bringing in the Positive with Additive Tapping

Additive tapping phrases
1. I wonder what it would be like if . . .
2. I can . . .
3. I am choosing to . . .
4. I am . . .

In the previous chapter, I talked about additive tapping, which is where we bring in the qualities that we desire more of. As discussed in chapter 2, one place you can look for inspiration is by accessing the NVC needs inventory using the link there. You'll find a very helpful tool to get clear on what it is you're wanting and needing in any situation (Rosenberg, 2003). This is also helpful for asking yourself what you want to bring in now that you've cleared the trauma. When you do additive tapping, start off by using these phrases in this order. With these phrases, you're moving progressively toward bringing what you want more of into the present moment as you move from the first statement through to the fourth statement. You're moving from possibility to certainty. After using these phrases to start, continue through the remaining tapping points as you invite in what you want. You can also incorporate these phrases while you're tapping through the rest of the points as well.

Additive tapping ideas	
Belonging	To be seen
Closeness	To be heard
Community	To be understood
Empathy	Trust
Respect/self-respect	Rest/sleep
Safety	Integrity
Security	Presence
Stability	Joy
Support	Choice

These are some of the additive tapping ideas for trauma from the needs inventory above. Do any of these resonate especially with you?

Additive Tapping Practice Process: Safety

Reductive tapping, which is what we did earlier to clear the charge and any additional emotional intensity, is very formulaic. Additive tapping is very much about art—sharing and naming whatever is coming up for you as you're going through the tapping process and inviting that in. You get to create and invite what it is you want. This is a sample process around safety to show another example of what this type of process can look like.

Go to www.bit.ly/PTSDHealing to access the additive tapping practice process: safety video. Use Messenger keyword: additive tapping.

Take a moment, with or without closed eyes, and tune into yourself. Notice how you're feeling emotionally and mentally. Once you have a sense of how you're feeling now, go through the tapping process below.

Additive Tapping Practice Round: Safety

1. **Left karate chop.** Say aloud, "I wonder what it would be like to feel safe in my body." **Deep inhale and a sigh.**

   Take your left hand and extend it in a karate chop as if you're about to chop wood. Take the four fingertips of the right hand and bring them to the karate chop area of the left hand. Make sure you're tapping on the meaty portion of the hand with your fingertips.

2. **Eyebrow.** Say aloud, "I can feel safe in my body." followed by a **deep inhale and a sigh.**

Bring the two index and the middle fingertips of both hands to the furry part of the eyebrows, right where they meet the nose. Tap there for a few moments.

3. **Side of the eye.** Say aloud, "I am choosing to feel safe in my body," followed by a **deep inhale and a sigh.**

    Then tap on the temples which are outside the eyebrows. You can feel there's a small indentation in the skull. Tap there.

4. **Cheekbone.** Say aloud, "I am safe in my body," followed by a **deep inhale and a sigh.**

    Tap on the cheekbones directly below the eyes. Your fingers should be directly in line with your eyes.

    After using the four statements we looked at earlier, now we'll use them in a little different way.

5. **Upper lip.** Say aloud, "I wonder what it would be like to make healthy boundaries," followed by a **deep inhale and a sigh.**

    With the fingertips of the index and middle fingers of one hand, tap below the nose in the crevice in the upper lip.

6. **Lower lip.** Say aloud, "I am making healthier boundaries," followed by a **deep inhale and a sigh.**

    Now tap in the crevice above the chin and below the bottom lip.

7. **Collarbone.** Say aloud, "When I make healthier boundaries, I respect myself," followed by a **deep inhale and a sigh.**

Now we're going to find the collarbone point. To me, this is the most difficult point to find. Feel your collarbones at the top of your chest. Below your collarbones is a hollow area. You can feel the sternum there as well, running up and down. Using your dominant hand, place your thumb on one side of it and your index and middle finger on the other side. You'll know it's the right place because it's soft there. Make sure that your thumb, index, and middle fingers are as close to your sternum as possible. Tap there for a moment.

8. **Heart.** Say aloud, "When I make healthier boundaries, I keep myself safe," followed by a **deep inhale and a sigh**.

   Place all four fingertips of your tapping hand right on your sternum above the heart. Tap there.

9. **Armpit.** Say aloud, "By making healthier boundaries, I build my self-worth," followed by a **deep inhale and a sigh**.

   Now tap on the armpit points. This is four inches below your armpits. Tap around in this area and see if there are any tender spots. If there are tender spots, tap right on them. If not, tap four inches below your armpits.

10. **Solar plexus.** Say aloud, "I take care of myself," followed by a **deep inhale and a sigh**. Let's say that again: "I take care of myself," followed by a **deep inhale and a sigh**.

    Find your solar plexus at the base of the ribs. Tap from the center of your bottom ribs out along the bottom ribs toward your sides. See if you can find any tender spots there. If you find any tender spots, tap right on them. If not, you can tap directly in line with the nipples.

11. **Left wrist.** Say aloud, "When I take care of myself, I give myself love and care," followed by a **deep inhale and a sigh.**

    Extend your left hand palm up toward the sky. Take the two fingertips of your right hand and tap on the center of the left wrist right where it meets the hand.

12. **Side of the left thumb.** Say aloud, "The more I offer love and care for myself, the safer I feel," followed by a **deep inhale and a sigh.**

    Then tap on the side of the left thumb, right by the nail, not on the nail or the underside of the finger. If you were to try to chop a piece of wood, this would be the part of your thumb that is facing toward the ceiling. Make sure you're using your fingertips.

    Make sure you're using your fingertips to tap directly on each point.

13. **Side of the left index finger.** Say aloud, "When I meet my own needs, others see how they can meet my needs too," followed by a **deep inhale and a sigh.**

    Tap on the side of the index finger on the same spot. Tap right on the side where the nail is but not on the nail.

14. **Side of the left middle finger.** Say aloud, "It feels so good and so kind to take care of myself," followed by a **deep inhale and a sigh.**

Repeat with the middle finger.

Keep your left hand still and just move your right hand. Leave the tapping fingers of the right hand extended as you rotate the tapping hand palm up toward the ceiling.

15. **Underside of the left ring finger.** Say aloud, "I feel safer being with myself," followed by a **deep inhale and a sigh.**

    Bring the fingertips onto the underside of your ring finger by the nail. If you were chopping wood with your left hand, it would be the side of your ring finger facing the ground.

16. **Underside of the left pinky finger.** Say aloud, "I feel safer in my body," followed by a **deep inhale and a sigh.**

    Continue tapping on the same spot on the pinky finger.

17. **Left karate chop.** Say aloud, "I breathe into the safety of being here right now." **Deep inhale into that sense of safety and a huge sigh.** "I breathe into the safety of being here right now." **Deep inhale, huge sigh.**

    Shake out your tapping hands. Notice how you're feeling after doing that additive tapping process.

What Does This Mean for PTSD Symptoms?

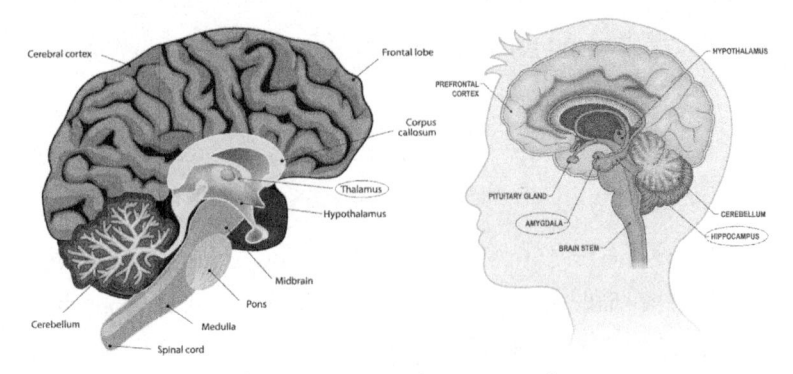

Figure 18. PTSD symptoms after processing the memories.

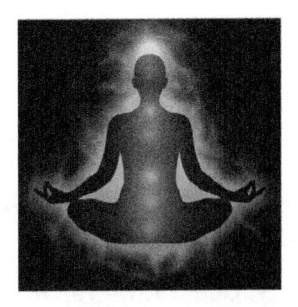

Figure 19. Safety and the chakras.

After you make your memory list and tap through the memories on it, how does that affect PTSD symptoms? From a biological perspective, trauma is caused by memories that are hanging around the amygdala that haven't yet moved into the hippocampus because of the substantial emotional charge (figure 18). The charge is what caused them to be retriggered by additional sensory input. By tapping on these memories, we're clearing the charge. These memories can then move into the hippocampus for long-term storage. As a result, you're not getting triggered by them in nearly the same way as before. This is because you've cleared the charge.

From an energetic perspective, since you've cleared the charge, you're able to be more present, as being present is less painful. You're less resistant to being present now. You're able to feel calmer because those memories aren't living in your system in the same way where you're feeling on edge and constantly attentive for danger.

As a result, we feel safer and more secure in life because you've cleared the trauma, allowing the root chakra to open up (figure 19). Being more present, calm, safe, and secure, we can show up better for ourselves and others.

PTSD Symptoms: An Energetic Perspective

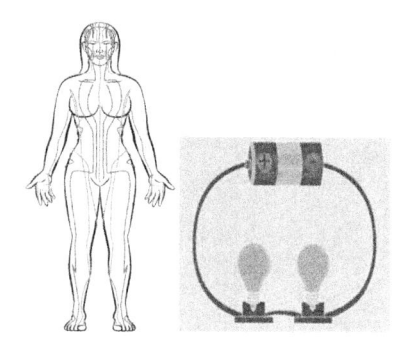

Figure 20. Unblock the energy circuit, give the system what it needs, and the body heals itself.

In the first chapter, we looked at the implications of trauma in the body as far as health and mental health outcomes. From this energetic perspective, we are clearing the blocks, allowing the energy to flow the way it naturally would. From an Eastern medicine and tapping perspective, the body has an innate intelligence. It will heal itself if it's given the tools and the fuel to do so. By getting the blocks out of the way, we are giving it just that. The body heals itself, and you might see that some other health issues decrease or are mitigated by the absence of the trauma. The trauma is no longer here in the same way it was before, and our health issues may have a significant shift as well. This is particularly likely with anxiety and depression according to the research data (Church & Brooks, 2014).

Does It Work? Case Study: Bill

What he said *before* he went through this process:	What he said *after* he went through this process:
Events during my day keep me awake.	I am not so anxious anymore.
I believe everything is my fault.	I don't get angry as fast and as intense as before.
I'm watchful, and I check multiple things to ensure everything is locked.	I am able to concentrate a lot more easily.
	My moods have been great and improved immensely.
	I don't let everything bother me anymore.
	I don't blame myself for everything.
	My relationship with others has greatly improved.
	I am able to sleep better.
	I was skeptical at first, but the results are amazing!

Figure 21. Bill's case study: before and after.

Let's take a look at this amazing case study with a client of mine who went through Clear My PTSD™, which is a course I created based on the same principles as this book (figure 21). For confidentiality purposes, we will call him Bill. He said that events during his day kept him awake at night, that he found that everything was his fault, and that he was watchful and hyper-vigilant in that he checked multiple things to ensure everything was locked. He was afraid of danger. After he went through this process, he said, "I'm not so anxious anymore. I don't get angry as fast or as intense as before. I'm able to concentrate a lot more and a lot more easily. My moods have been great and improved immensely. I don't let everything bother me anymore. I don't blame myself for everything. My relationship with others has greatly improved, and I'm able to sleep better as well. I was skeptical at first, but the results are amazing."

Bill's Scores

Issue	Before Clear My PTSD	After 8 weeks of Clear My PTSD
PTSD	85/100	39/100
Depression	73/100	11/100
Anxiety	55/100	8/100

Figure 22. Bill's scores: before and after.

Bill took real clinical assessments before going through the course. These are Bill's scores. After going through the course, his PTSD decreased from 85/100 to 39/100. His depression dropped from 73/100 to 11/100, and his anxiety plummeted from 55/100 to 8/100. He did this in just 14 hours by following the exact processes and principles that I have shown you in this book.

Go to www.bit.ly/PTSDHealing to access the cheat sheet and summary for chapter 3. Use Messenger keyword: chapter three cheat sheet.

Chapter Three Brief Summary

- Trauma impacts our sense of safety. Therefore, when healing trauma, creating and maintaining safety is a key component of the process.
- We create safety through resourcing meditation. Over time and during the trauma healing process, we retrain our system to experience safety using this meditation.
- The window of tolerance is another key tool in keeping ourselves safe during trauma healing.
- We stay in the window by doing the trauma healing progressively, rather than overloading our system by doing it all at once.
- We do the healing progressively by telling the story until we reach certain degrees of intensity, each time Tapping through the intensity and then doing the resourcing meditation before continuing.

To learn how to create safety for yourself so you can effectively move through the trauma and PTSD healing process, join us for the Clear My PTSD Healing Accelerator at www.ClearMyPTSD.com/course

Implementing the Trauma Healing Blueprint

Rumi said, "The wound is the place where the Light enters you." Let's heal the wounds so you can bring in more and more light.

A. **Pre-Trauma Healing Preparation**

    1. Create and record your own resourcing meditation (chapter 3).

        a. Begin practicing this daily until you notice a change in your sense of embodied safety.

        b. Move onto the Trauma Healing Process below at your own pace. This might mean you decide to start working with your trauma today, a week from now, a month from now, in six months, a year, or two years. It all depends on when you feel safer and ready to begin the work.

    2. Learn and practice the tapping points using the methods in chapter two. Become familiar with the points.

B. **The Trauma Healing Process**

    3. Create your list of memories affecting your experience of trauma and PTSD. List and rank the memories as described in chapter 3.

    4. Begin to work through the traumatic memories from most intense to least intense using the 3/10, 6/10, 10/10 approach outlined in chapter 3. Continue this process with all of the memories on your list.

C. Self-Care

    5. While you're working through the trauma, implement one self-care process in your daily routine as described in chapter 1. If this is too difficult to implement because of the time commitment while you're also doing trauma work, implement one self-care item per day after you finish working through your memories.

        a. After you incorporate one per day, see if you can incorporate more. For example: meditation, an Epsom salt bath, and some form of exercise in one day.

D. Managing Daily Emotions

    6. Learn and practice the skills in chapter one and two to manage your daily emotions. Take photos or retype/rewrite the aura process and violet flame process so you can have access to them on your phone.

        a. When you notice yourself having difficult emotions, you can use the aura process (chapter 1) or tapping (chapter 2). If the emotion doesn't fully integrate immediately, repeat the process, noticing how you feel after each repetition.

        b. Use the violet flame process only after you've fully integrated and worked through whatever difficult emotion you were experiencing.

Reviews

Did you find this book helpful?

If you've found this book helpful, it would be wonderful if you could leave a review on Amazon. I really appreciate hearing how this book has impacted you, and other people on their own healing path will as well.

Thank you!

RESOURCE LIST

Below is the quick access guide for the resources used throughout this book. To access all resources, enter the listed keyword into Facebook Messenger at www.bit.ly/PTSDHealing unless otherwise stated.

Introduction

To get a sense of how you're doing with PTSD, access the PTSD checkup using Messenger keyword: PTSD Checkup.

Join our supportive community of folks like you who are healing their trauma in the David Redbord, Transformation from Within Facebook Group at http://bit.ly/PTSDFBGroup and Like the David Redbord Facebook Page at http://bit.ly/PTSDFBPage.

Chapter One

Gain an understanding of how your trauma history may be impacting your health with the ACE questionnaire. Use Messenger keyword: ACE questionnaire.

Strengthen Your Identity

Learn about how you interact with the world and make decisions with the Myers-Briggs personality test. Use Messenger keyword: Myers-Briggs.

Understand your strengths and how you can use them even more with the VIA strengths survey. Use Messenger keyword: strengths survey.

Clarify your path toward more well-being from a personality standpoint with the Enneagram. Use Messenger keyword: Enneagram.

Mindfulness Meditation

Practice becoming present through mindfulness with the mindfulness meditation exercise video and handout. Use Messenger keyword: mindfulness meditation.

Working with Emotions

Integrate difficult emotions using the the aura process video and handout. Use Messenger keyword: aura process.

For very stubborn, heavy energy use the violet flame process video and handout. Use Messenger keyword: violet flame.

Cheat Sheet

For the full cheat sheet and chapter summary, use Messenger keyword: chapter one cheat sheet.

Chapter Two

Tapping Resources

To learn the tapping points used throughout this book, use the tapping points introduction video and handout. Use Messenger keyword: tapping points introduction.

To strengthen the impact of all your tapping work, check out the tapping with breath and sound video and handout. Use Messenger keyword: breath and sound.

Integrate difficult emotions with Tapping using the reductive tapping practice round video and handout. Use Messenger keyword: full practice round.

Getting Clear On What to Tap On

Clarify your feelings using the feelings inventory. Use Messenger keyword: feelings inventory.

Invite in more of what you want using the needs inventory. Use Messenger keyword: needs inventory.

Cheat Sheet

For the full cheat sheet and chapter summary, use Messenger keyword: chapter two cheat sheet.

Chapter 3

Creating Safety

To create a sense of safety for yourself, access the resourcing meditation video, template, and script. Use Messenger keyword: resourcing meditation

Trauma Healing Roadmap

To create your individualized trauma healing roadmap, use the traumatic memory list template. Use Messenger keyword: traumatic memory list

Bringing in the Positive

To learn how to bring in positive beliefs with Tapping, check out the the additive tapping practice process: safety video. Use Messenger keyword: additive tapping.

Cheat Sheet

For the full cheat sheet and chapter summary. Use Messenger keyword: chapter three cheat sheet.

WORKS CITED

About the CDC-Kaiser ACE Study. (2019). Retrieved from https://www.cdc.gov/violenceprevention/childabuseandneglect/acestudy/about.html

Behavioral Risk Factor Surveillance System ACE Data. (2019). Retrieved from https://www.cdc.gov/violenceprevention/childabuseandneglect/acestudy/ace-brfss.html

Call, B. R. (2010). *Crafter's devotional: 365 days of tips, tricks, and techniques for unlocking your creative spirit.* Gloucester, Mass: Quarry.

Church et al. (2013) Psychological trauma symptom improvement in veterans using emotional freedom techniques: A randomized controlled trial. *The Journal of Nervous and Mental Disease,* 201(2), 153–160.

Church, D. (2013). *The EFT manual: Third edition.* Santa Rosa, CA: Energy Psychology Press.

Church, D. (2017). *Eft for ptsd.* Fulton, CA: Energy Psychology Press

Church, D., Piña, O., Reategui, C., & Brooks, A. J. (2012). Single session reduction of the intensity of traumatic memories in abused adolescents: A randomized controlled trial. *Traumatology, 18*(3), 73-79. doi:10.1177/1534765611426788

Church, D., Stapleton, P., Mollon, P., Feinstein, D., Boath, E., Mackay, D., & Sims, R. (2018). Guidelines for the Treatment of PTSD Using Clinical EFT (Emotional Freedom Techniques). *Healthcare (Basel, Switzerland), 6*(4), 146. doi:10.3390/healthcare6040146

Cognitive Processing Therapy (CPT). (2017). Retrieved from https://www.apa.org/ptsd-guideline/treatments/cognitive-processing-therapy

Craig, G., & Fowlie, A. (1995). Emotional Freedom Techniques: The manual. Sea Ranch, CA: Gary Craig.

David, M. (1991). *Nourishing wisdom: A mind/body approach to nutrition and well-being.* New York: Bell Tower.

Dawson, K. & Allenby, S. (2010). *Matrix reimprinting using eft.* London, UK: Hay House.

Dawson, K. & Marillat, K. (2014). *Transform your beliefs, transform your life.* London, UK: Hay House UK Ltd.

Ellis, K. (2014). *Worrier to warrior: Conquer anxiety & panic attacks program.* Scottsdale, AZ: The Healing Quest Publishing

Eye Movement Desensitization and Reprocessing (EMDR) Therapy (2017). Retrieved from https://www.apa.org/ptsd-guideline/treatments/eye-movement-reprocessing

Felitti, V. J., Andra, R. F., & Nordenberg, D., Williamson, D. F., Spitz, A. M., Edwards, V., Koss, M. P., & Marks, J. S. (1998). Relationship of childhood abuse and household dysfunction to many of the leading causes of death in adults: The adverse childhood experiences (ACE) study. *American Journal of Preventative Medicine, 14*(4), 245-258. https://doi.org/10.1016/S0749-3797(98)00017-8

Gallo, F. P. (2007). *Energy tapping for trauma: Rapid relief from post-traumatic stress using energy psychology.* Oakland, CA: New Harbinger Publications, Inc.

Gurret, J. M., Caufour, C., Palmer-Hoffman, J., & Church, D. (2012). Post-earthquake rehabilitation of clinical PTSD in Haitian seminarians. *Energy Psychology: Theory, Research, and Treatment, 4*(2), 33-40.

Harrington, R. (2013). *Stress, health & well-being: Thriving in the 21st century.* Belmont, CA: Wadsworth Cengage Learning.

Hartmann, S. (2003). *Adventures in eft: Sixth edition.* Eastbourne, UK: Gardners Books.

Heller, L., & LaPierre, A. (2012). *Healing developmental trauma: How early trauma affects self-regulation, self-image, and the capacity for relationship.* Berkeley, CA: North Atlantic Books

Jalāl al-Dīn Rūmī., & Barks, C. (1996). *The essential Rumi.* 1st HarperCollins paperback ed. San Francisco, CA: Harper.

Judith, A., & Jennings, L. 2016. *Eastern body, western mind: Psychology and the chakra system as a path to the self.* Old Saybrook, Conn: Tantor Media.

Kabat-Zinn, J., & University of Massachusetts Medical Center/Worcester. (1991). *Full catastrophe living: Using the wisdom of your body and mind to face stress, pain, and illness.* New York, N.Y: Dell Pub., a division of Bantam Doubleday Dell Pub. Group.

Kar, N. (2011). Cognitive behavioral therapy for the treatment of post-traumatic stress disorder: a review. *Neuropsychiatric disease and treatment, 7*, 167–181. doi:10.2147/NDT.S10389

Keirsey, D., & Bates, M. M. (1978). *Please understand me: Character & temperament types.* Del Mar, CA: Prometheus Nemesis.

Levine, P. A. (2012). *Healing trauma: A pioneering program for restoring the wisdom of your body.* Boulder, CO: Sounds True, Inc.

National Collaborating Centre for Mental Health (UK). (2005). Post-traumatic stress disorder: The management of ptsd in adults and children in primary and secondary care. *NICE Clinical Guidelines, 26*(2). https://www.ncbi.nlm.nih.gov/books/NBK56506/

Nemiro, A., Papworth, S. (2015). Efficacy of two evidence-based therapies, Emotional Freedom Techniques (EFT) and Cognitive Behavioral Therapy (CBT) for the treatment of gender violence in the Congo: A randomized controlled trial. *Energy Psychology: Theory, Research, & Treatment*, 7(2), 13-25. doi:10.9769/EPJ.2015.11.1.AN

Ogden, P., Minton, K., & Pain, C. (2006). *Trauma and the body: A sensorimotor approach to psychotherapy*. New York: W.W. Norton.

Ortner, N. (2014). *Tapping solution: A revolutionary system for stress-free living*. Carlsbad, CA: Hay House, Inc.

Peterson, C., & Seligman, M. E. P. (2004). *Character strengths and virtues: A handbook and classification*. Washington, DC: American Psychological Association.

Prolonged Exposure (PE). (2017). Retrieved from https://www.apa.org/ptsd-guideline/treatments/prolonged-exposure

Scruton, R. (1996). The eclipse of listening. *The New Criterion*, 15(3), 5-13.

Pyle, K. (1918). *Mother's nursery tales*. New York, NY: E.P. Dutton & Company

Riedl, M. (2006). *Yoni massage: Awakening female sexual energy*. Rochester, VT: Inner Traditions International.

Riso, D. R., & Hudson, R. (1999). *The wisdom of the enneagram: The complete guide to psychological and spiritual growth for the nine personality types*. New York, NY: Bantam Books.

Rosenberg, M. B. (2003). *Nonviolent communication: A language of life*. Encinitas, CA: PuddleDancer Press.

Russ, S. W., & Wallace, C. E. (2013). Pretend play and creative processes. *American Journal of Play, 6*(1), 136-148.

Schulte, B. (2014). *Overwhelmed: How to work, love and play when no one has the time.* New York: Picador.

Seltzer, L. F. (2016). You only get more of what you resist—why?. Retrieved from https://www.psychologytoday.com/us/blog/evolution-the-self/201606/you-only-get-more-what-you-resist-why

Siegel, Daniel J. (2012). *Developing Mind, Second Edition: How Relationships and the Brain Interact to Shape Who We Are.* Guilford Press.

Singh, R. (2015). *Miracles with eft: Free yourself from mental, emotional and physical pain in minutes.* Haryana, India: Hay House, Inc

Solomon, K. (2007). *Tapping into wellness: Using eft to clear emotional & physical pain & illness.* Woodbury, MN: Llewellyn Publications.

Spiers, T. (2001). *Trauma: A practitioner's guide to counseling.* Hove, UK: Routledge.

Tedeschi, R., & Calhoun, L. (1996). The posttraumatic growth inventory: Measuring the positive legacy of trauma. *Journal of Traumatic Stress, 9,* 455–471. doi: 10.1002/jts.2490090305.

van der Kolk, B. A. (2014). *The body keeps the score: Brain, mind, and body in the healing of trauma.* New York: Viking.

Weinhold, B. K., & Weinhold, J. B. (2017). *How to break free of the drama triangle and victim consciousness.* Asheville, NC: CICRCL Press.

Printed in Great Britain
by Amazon